Biotechnology
Fourth Edition

Biotechnology will undoubtedly be the major technology of the twenty-first century. It concerns the practical application of biological organisms or their various components to the benefit of humankind, and spans a multitude of modern and traditional industries. The rise of genetic engineering, genomics and proteomics and the creation of transgenic crops and animals have revolutionised activities as varied as brewing beer and the treatment of sewage and waste water, to drug development and agriculture.

In this expanded fourth edition of his popular textbook, John Smith once again demystifies biotechnology, and especially genetic manipulation, clearly and accessibly, explaining the history, techniques and applications of modern biotechnology for students and the general reader. All aspects of biotechnology are covered and a positive stance is taken concerning the potential benefits to human society. In this edition, greater emphasis is given to the public perception of biotechnology and the ethical and safety questions raised.

JOHN E. SMITH is Emeritus Professor of Applied Microbiology in the Department of Bioscience, University of Strathclyde, Glasgow and Chief Scientific Adviser to Myco-Biotech Ltd, Singapore.

The **Studies in Biology** series is published in association with the Institute of Biology (London, UK). The series provides short, affordable and very readable textbooks aimed primarily at undergraduate biology students. Each book offers either an introduction to a broad area of biology (e.g. *Introductory Microbiology*) or a more in-depth treatment of a particular system of specific topic (e.g. *Photosynthesis*). All of the subjects and systems covered are selected on the basis that all undergraduate students will study them at some point during their biology degree courses.

Titles available in this series

An Introduction to Genetic Engineering, 2nd edition, D. S. T. Nicholl

Introductory Microbiology, J. Heritage, E. G. V. Evans and R. A. Killington

An Introduction to Parasitology, B. E. Matthews

Photosynthesis, 6th edition. D. O. Hall and K. K. Rao

Microbiology in Action, J. Heritage, E. G. V. Evans and R. A. Killington

Essentials of Animal Behaviour, P. J. B. Slater

An Introduction to the Invertebrates, J. Moore

Nerve and Muscle, 3rd edition, R. D. Keynes and D. J. Aidley

Biotechnology, 4th edition, J. E. Smith

Biotechnology
Fourth Edition

John E. Smith
Emeritus Professor of Applied Microbiology,
University of Strathclyde, Glasgow and
Chief Scientific Adviser to MycoBiotech Ltd, Singapore

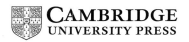

PUBLISHED BY THE PRESS SYNDICATE OF THE UNIVERSITY OF CAMBRIDGE
The Pitt Building, Trumpington Street, Cambridge, United Kingdom

CAMBRIDGE UNIVERSITY PRESS
The Edinburgh Building, Cambridge, CB2 2RU, UK
40 West 20th Street, New York, NY 10011–4211, USA
477 Williamstown Road, Port Melbourne, VIC 3207, Australia
Ruiz de Alarcón 13, 28014 Madrid, Spain
Dock House, The Waterfront, Cape Town 8001, South Africa

http://www.cambridge.org

First published 2004

Printed in the United Kingdom at the University Press, Cambridge

Typefaces Adobe Garamond 11/13 pt. and Frutiger   *System* LaTeX 2$_\varepsilon$ [TB]

A catalogue record for this book is available from the British Library

Library of Congress Cataloguing in Publication Data
Smith, John E.
Biotechnology/John E. Smith – 4th ed.
    p.   cm. – (Studies in biology)
Includes bibliographical references and index.
ISBN 0 521 83332 9 (hbk.) – ISBN 0 521 54077 1 (pbk.)
1. Biotechnology.   I. Title.   II. Series.
TP248.2.S66   2004
660.6 – dc22   2003065269

ISBN 0 521 83332 9 hardback
ISBN 0 521 54077 1 paperback

The publisher has used its best endeavours to ensure that the URLs for external websites
referred to in this book are correct and active at the time of going to press. However, the
publisher has no responsibility for the websites and can make no guarantee that a site will
remain live or that the content is or will remain appropriate.

I dedicate this fourth edition to my
wife, Evelyn, for her patience and support.

Contents

Preface

Biotechnology is, in essence, the deciphering and use of biological knowledge. It is highly multidisciplinary since it has its foundations in many disciplines, including biology, microbiology, biochemistry, molecular biology, genetics, chemistry and chemical and process engineering. It may also be viewed as a series of enabling technologies that involve the practical application of organisms (especially microorganisms) or their cellular components to manufacturing and service industries and environmental management. Historically, biotechnology was an artisanal skill rather than a science, exemplified by the manufacture of wines, beers, cheese, etc., where the techniques of manufacture were well worked out and reproducible, while the biological mechanisms were not understood. As the scientific basis of these biotechnology processes has developed, this has led to more efficient manufacturing of the traditional processes that still represent the major financial rewards of biotechnology. Modern biotechnological processes have generated a wide range of new and novel products, including antibiotics, recombinant proteins and vaccines, and monoclonal antibodies, the production of which has been optimised by improved fermentation practices. Biotechnology has been further revolutionised by a range of new molecular innovations, allowing unprecedented molecular changes to be made to living organisms. Genomics and proteomics are now heralding a new age of biotechnology, especially in the areas of human health and food production. In the environment, biotechnology innovations are creating major advances in water and land management and also remediating the pollution guaranteed by over-industrialisation.

Some of the new aspects of biotechnology, such as genetic engineering, have aroused certain social sensitivities of an ethical, moral and political character.

Regulatory authorities throughout the world are now examining the implications of these new and revolutionary techniques. It is hoped that common sense will prevail.

Undoubtedly, modern biotechnology can only maximise its full potential to benefit mankind through achieving a basis of public understanding and awareness and knowledge of the technologies. Participating scientists must learn to communicate openly with the public and attempt to demystify the complex nature of living systems. By doing so they will generate a greater level of confidence and trust between the scientific community and the public at large.

This expanded fourth edition of *Biotechnology* is again aimed at giving an integrated overview of its complex, multifaceted and often ill-judged subjects and, for some young readers, at pointing the way forward to exciting, satisfying and rewarding careers. Biotechnology will undoubtedly be the major technology of the twenty-first century.

I am again deeply indebted to Miss Elizabeth Clements for her skilful processing of the manuscript.

1

The nature of biotechnology

1.1 Introduction

Major events in human history have, to a large extent, been driven by technology. Improved awareness of agriculture and metalworking brought mankind out of the Stone Age, while in the nineteenth century, the Industrial Revolution created a multitude of machinery together with ever-increasingly larger cities. The twentieth century was undoubtedly the age of chemistry and physics, spawning huge industrial activities such as petrochemicals, pharmaceuticals, fertilisers, the atom bomb, transmitters, the laser and microchips. However, there can be little doubt that the huge understanding of the fundamentals of life processes achieved in the latter part of the twentieth century will ensure that the twenty-first century will be dominated by biology and the associated technologies.

Societal changes are increasingly driven by science and technology. Currently, the impact of new biological developments must be absorbed not just by a minority (the scientists) but also by large numbers (the general public). If this does not happen the majority will be alienated. It is increasingly important to ensure a broad understanding of what bioscience and its related technologies will involve, and especially what the consequences will be of accepting or rejecting the new technical innovations.

The following chapters will examine how the new biotechnologists are: developing new therapies and cures for many human and animal diseases; designing diagnostic tests for increasing disease prevention and pollution control; improving many aspects of plant and animal agriculture; cleaning and improving the environment; and designing clean industrial manufacturing processes. Undoubtedly, biotechnology can be seen to be the most innovative technology that mankind has witnessed.

While biotechnology will undoubtedly offer major opportunities to human development (nutrition, medicine, industry), it cannot be denied that it is creating social/ethical apprehensions because of considered dangers to human rights that improper use could create. The advancement of genetic engineering, and especially the ramifications of the Human Genome Project, are achieving unique importance.

1.2 What is biotechnology?

There is little doubt that modern biology is the most diversified of all the natural sciences, exhibiting a bewildering array of subdisciplines: microbiology, plant and animal anatomy, biochemistry, immunology, cell biology, molecular biology, plant and animal physiology, morphogenesis, systematics, ecology, genetics and many others. The increasing diversity of modern biology has been derived primarily from the largely post-war introduction into biology of other scientific disciplines, such as physics, chemistry and mathematics, which have made possible the description of life processes at the cellular and molecular level. In the last two decades, well over 20 Nobel prizes have been awarded for discoveries in these fields of study.

This newly acquired biological knowledge has already made vastly important contributions to the health and welfare of mankind. Yet few people fully recognise that the life sciences affect over 30% of global economic turnover by way of health care, food and energy, agriculture and forestry, and that this economic impact will grow as biotechnology provides new ways of influencing raw material processing. Biotechnology will increasingly affect the efficiency of all fields involving the life sciences and it is now realistically accepted that, by the early twenty-first century, it will be contributing many trillions of pounds to world markets.

In the following chapters, biotechnology will be shown to cover a multitude of different applications, ranging from the very simple and traditional, such as the production of beers, wines and cheeses, to highly complex molecular processes such as the use of recombinant DNA technologies to yield new drugs or to introduce new traits into commercial crops and animals. The association of old traditional industries such as brewing with modern genetic engineering is gaining in momentum and it is not for nothing that industrial giants such as Guinness, Carlsberg and Bass are heavily involved in biotechnology research. Biotechnology is developing at a phenomenal pace and will increasingly be

Table 1.1. Some selected definitions of biotechnology

The application of biological organisms, systems or processes to manufacturing and service industries.

The integrated use of biochemistry, microbiology and engineering sciences in order to achieve technological (industrial) application capabilities of microorganisms, cultured tissue cells and parts thereof.

A technology using biological phenomena for copying and manufacturing various kinds of useful substances.

The application of scientific and engineering principles to the processing of materials by biological agents to provide goods and services.

The science of the production processes based on the action of microorganisms and their active components and of production processes involving the use of cells and tissues from higher organisms. Medical technology, agriculture and traditional crop breeding are not generally regarded as biotechnology.

Really no more than a name given to a set of techniques and processes.

The use of living organisms and their components in agriculture, food production and other industrial processes.

The deciphering and use of biological knowledge.

The application of our knowledge and understanding of biology to meet practical needs.

seen as a necessary part of the advance of modern life and not simply a way to make money!

While biotechnology has been defined in many forms (Table 1.1), in essence it implies the use of microbial, animal or plant cells or enzymes to synthesise, break down or transform materials.

The European Federation of Biotechnology (EFB) considers biotechnology as 'the integration of natural sciences and organisms, cells, parts thereof, and molecular analogues for products and services'. The aims of this Federation are:

(1) to advance biotechnology for the public benefit;
(2) to promote awareness, communication and collaboration in all fields of biotechnology;
(3) to provide governmental and supranational bodies with information and informed opinions on biotechnology;
(4) to promote public understanding of biotechnology.

The EFB definition is applicable to both 'traditional or old' and 'new or modern' biotechnology. Traditional biotechnology refers to the conventional

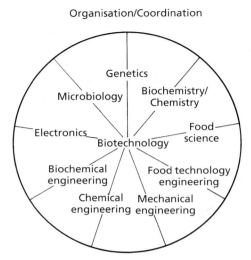

Fig. 1.1   The interdisciplinary nature of biotechnology (from Higgins *et al.*, 1985).

techniques which have been used for many centuries to produce beer, wine, cheese and many other foods, while 'new' biotechnology embraces all methods of genetic modification by recombinant DNA and cell fusion techniques together with the modern developments of 'traditional' biotechnological processes.

The difficulties of defining biotechnology and the resulting misunderstandings have led some to suggest the abandonment of the term 'biotechnology' as too general and the replacement of it by the precise term of whatever specific technology or application is being used.

Unlike a single scientific discipline, biotechnology can draw upon a wide array of relevant fields, such as microbiology, biochemistry, molecular biology, cell biology, immunology, protein engineering, enzymology, classified breeding techniques, and the full range of bioprocess technologies (Fig. 1.1). Biotechnology is not itself a product or range of products like microelectronics: rather it should be regarded as a range of enabling technologies which will find significant application in many industrial sectors. As will be seen in later sections, it is a technology in search of new applications, and the main benefits lie in the future. New biotechnological processes will, in many instances, function at low temperature, will consume little energy, and will rely mainly on inexpensive substrates for biosynthesis.

As stated by McCormick (1996), a former editor of the *Journal of Bio/Technology*, 'There is no such thing as biotechnology, there are biotechnologies.

Table 1.2. Historical development of biotechnology

Biotechnological production of foods and beverages
Sumerians and Babylonians were drinking beer by 6000 BC; Egyptians were baking
leavened bread by 4000 BC; wine was known in the Near East by the time of the
book of Genesis. Microorganisms were first seen in the seventeenth century by
Anton van Leeuwenhoek, who developed the simple microscope, and the
fermentative ability of microorganisms was demonstrated between 1857 and 1876
by Pasteur – **the father of biotechnology**. Cheese production has ancient origins,
as does mushroom cultivation.

Biotechnological processes initially developed under non-sterile conditions
Ethanol, acetic acid, butanol and acetone were produced by the end of the
nineteenth century by open microbial fermentation processes. Waste-water
treatment and municipal composting of solid wastes created the largest
fermentation capacity practised throughout the world.

Introduction of sterility to biotechnological processes
In the 1940s, complicated engineering techniques were applied to the mass
cultivation of microorganisms to exclude contaminating microorganisms, e.g. in the
cultivation of antibiotics, amino acids, organic acids, enzymes, steroids,
polysaccharides, vaccines and monoclonal antibodies.

Applied genetics and recombinant DNA technology
Traditional strain improvement of important industrial organisms has long been
practised; recombinant DNA techniques, together with protoplast fusion, allow new
programming of the biological properties of organisms.

There is no biotechnology industry; there are industries that depend on
biotechnologies for new products and competitive advantage.'

It should be recognised that biotechnology is not something new but something which represents a developing and expanding series of technologies
dating back (in many cases) thousands of years, when humans first began
unwittingly to use microbes to produce foods and beverages like bread and
beer and to modify plants and animals through progressive selection for desired
traits. Biotechnology encompasses many traditional processes such as brewing, baking, winemaking, production of cheese and oriental foods such as soy
sauce and tempeh, and sewage treatment, where the use of microorganisms
has been developed somewhat empirically over countless years (Table 1.2). It
is only relatively recently that these processes have been subjected to rigorous

scientific scrutiny and analysis; even so it will surely take some time, if at all, for modern scientifically based practices to fully replace traditional empiricism.

The new biotechnology revolution began in the 1970s and early 1980s when scientists learned to alter precisely the genetic constitution of living organisms by processes outside of traditional breeding practices. This 'genetic engineering' has had profound impact on almost all areas of traditional biotechnology and has further permitted breakthroughs in medicine and agriculture, in particular, that would be impossible by traditional breeding approaches. Some of the most exciting advances will be in the development of new pharmaceutical drugs and therapies aimed at improving treatments to many diseases, and in producing healthier foods, selective pesticides, and innovative environmental technologies.

There is also a considerable danger that biotechnology will be viewed as a coherent, unified body of scientific and engineering knowledge and thinking to be applied in a coherent and logical manner. This is not so; the range of biological, chemical and engineering disciplines that are involved have varying degrees of application to the industrial scene.

Traditional biotechnology has established a huge and expanding world market and, in monetary terms, represents a major part of *all* biotechnology financial profits. 'New' aspects of biotechnology founded in recent advances in molecular biology, genetic engineering and fermentation process technology are now increasingly finding wide industrial application. A width of relevant biological and engineering knowledge and expertise is ready to be put to productive use; however, the rate at which it will be applied will depend less on scientific or technical considerations and more on such factors as adequate investment by the relevant industries, improved systems of biological patenting, marketing skills, the economics of the new methods in relation to currently employed technologies, and – possibly of most importance – public perception and acceptance.

The present industrial activities to be most affected will include human and animal food production, provision of chemical feedstocks to replace petrochemical sources, alternative energy sources, waste recycling, pollution control, agriculture, aquaculture and forestry. From a medical dimension, biotechnology will focus on the development of biological compounds rather than on chemical compounds. Use will be made of proteins, hormones and related substances that occur in the living system or even in those that are created *in vitro*. The new techniques will also revolutionise many aspects of medicine, veterinary sciences, and pharmaceutics. The recent mapping of the human genome must be recognised as one of the most significant breakthroughs in human history.

Many biotechnological industries will be based largely on renewable and recyclable materials and so can be adapted to the needs of a society in which energy is ever increasingly expensive and scarce. In many ways, biotechnology is a series of embryonic technologies and will require much skilful control of its development, but the potentials are vast and diverse, and undoubtedly will play an increasingly important part in many future industrial processes.

1.3   Biotechnology: an interdisciplinary pursuit

Biotechnology is a priori an interdisciplinary pursuit. In recent decades a characteristic feature of the development of science and technology has been the increasing resort to multidisciplinary strategies for the solution of various problems. This has led to the emergence of new interdisciplinary areas of study, with the eventual crystallisation of new disciplines with identifiable characteristic concepts and methodologies.

Chemical engineering and biochemistry are two well-recognised examples of disciplines that have done much to clarify our understanding of chemical processes and the biochemical bases of biological systems.

The term '*multidisciplinary*' describes a quantitative extension of approaches to problems which commonly occur within a given area. It involves the marshalling of concepts and methodologies from a number of separate disciplines and applying them to a specific problem in another area. In contrast, '*interdisciplinary*' application occurs when the blending of ideas which occur during multidisciplinary cooperation leads to the crystallisation of a new disciplinary area with its own concepts and methodologies. In practice, multidisciplinary enterprises are almost invariably mission-orientated. However, when true interdisciplinary synthesis occurs, the new area will open up a novel spectrum of investigations. Many aspects of biotechnology have arisen through the interaction between various parts of biology and engineering.

A biotechnologist can utilise techniques derived from chemistry, microbiology, biochemistry, chemical engineering and computer science (Fig. 1.1). The main objectives will be the innovation, development and optimal operation of processes in which biochemical catalysis has a fundamental and irreplaceable role. Biotechnologists must also aim to achieve a close working cooperation with experts from other related fields such as medicine, nutrition, the pharmaceutical and chemical industries, environmental protection and waste process technology.

The industrial application of biotechnology will increasingly rest upon each of the contributing disciplines in order to understand the technical language

Table 1.3. Types of companies involved with biotechnology

Category	Biotechnology involvement
Therapeutics	Pharmaceutical products for the cure or control of human diseases, including antibiotics, vaccines and gene therapy.
Diagnostics	Clinical testing and diagnosis, food, environment, agriculture.
Agriculture/forestry/ horticulture	Novel crops or animal varieties, pesticides.
Food	Wide range of food products, fertilisers, beverages, ingredients.
Environment	Waste treatment, bioremediation, energy production.
Chemical intermediates	Reagents including enzymes, DNA/RNA and speciality chemicals.
Equipment	Hardware, bioreactors, software and consumables supporting biotechnology.

of the others and, above all, to understand the potential as well as the limitations of the other areas. For instance, for the fermentation bio-industries the traditional education for chemical engineers and industrial plant designers has not normally included biological processes. The nature of the materials required, the reactor vessels (bioreactors) and the operating conditions are so different that it requires complete retraining.

Biotechnology is a demanding industry that requires a skilled workforce and a supportive public to ensure continued growth. Economies that encourage public understanding and provide a competent labour force should achieve long-term benefits from biotechnology. The main types of companies involved with biotechnology can be placed in seven categories (Table 1.3).

A key factor in the distinction between biology and biotechnology is their scale of operation. The biologist usually works in the range between nanograms and milligrams. The biotechnologist working on the production of vaccines may be satisfied with milligram yields, but in many other projects aims are at kilograms or tonnes. Thus, one of the main aspects of biotechnology consists of scaling-up biological processes.

Many present-day biotechnological processes have their origins in ancient and traditional fermentations such as the brewing of beer and the manufacture of bread, cheese, yoghurt, wine and vinegar. However, it was the discovery of antibiotics in 1929 and their subsequent large-scale production in the 1940s

Table 1.4. World markets for biological products, 1981

Product	Sales ($ million)
Alcoholic beverages	23 000
Cheese	14 000
Antibiotics	4 500
Penicillins	500
Tetracyclines	500
Cephalosporins	450
Diagnostic tests	2 000
Immunoassay	400
Monoclonal	5
Seeds	1 400
High fructose syrups	800
Amino acids	750
Baker's yeast	540
Steroids	500
Vitamins, all	330
C	200
B_{12}	14
Citric acid	210
Enzymes	200
Vaccines	150
Human serum albumin	125
Insulin	100
Urokinase	50
Human factor VIII protein	40
Human growth hormone	35
Microbial pesticides	12

that created the greatest advances in fermentation technology. Since then we have witnessed a phenomenal development in this technology, not only in the production of antibiotics but also of many other useful, simple or complex biochemical products, for example organic acids, polysaccharides, enzymes, vaccines, hormones, etc. (Table 1.4). Inherent in the development of fermentation processes is the growing close relationship between the biochemist, the microbiologist and the chemical engineer. Thus, biotechnology is not a sudden discovery but rather a coming of age of a technology that was initiated several decades ago. Looking to the future, *The Economist*, when reporting on this new technology, stated that it may launch 'an industry as characteristic of the twenty-first century as those based on physics and chemistry have been of the twentieth century'.

If it is accepted that biotechnology has its roots in distant history and has large successful industrial outlets, why then has there been such public awareness of this subject in recent years? Undoubtedly the main dominating reason must derive from the rapid advances in molecular biology, in particular recombinant DNA technology, which is giving humans dominance over nature. By these new techniques (to be discussed in Chapters 3, 8, 10) it is possible to manipulate directly the heritable material (DNA) of cells between different types of organisms *in vitro*, creating new hybrid DNA molecules not previously known to exist in nature. The potential of this series of techniques first developed in academic laboratories is now being rapidly exploited in industry, agriculture and medicine. While the benefits are immense, the inherent dangers of tampering with nature must always be appreciated and respected.

While in theory the technology is available to transfer a particular gene from any organism into any other organism, microorganism, plant or animal (Chapter 3), in actual practice there are numerous constraining factors, such as which genes to be cloned, and how they can be selected. The single most limiting factor in the application of genetic engineering is the dearth of basic scientific knowledge of gene structure and function.

The developments of biotechnology are proceeding at a speed similar to those of micro-electronics in the mid-1970s. Although the analogy is tempting, any expectations that biotechnology will develop commercially at the same spectacular rate should be tempered with considerable caution. While the potential of 'new' biotechnology cannot be doubted, a meaningful commercial realisation is now only slowly occurring and will accelerate throughout the twenty-first century. New biotechnology will have a considerable impact across all industrial uses of the life sciences. In each case the relative merits of competing means of production will influence the economics of a biotechnological route. Biotechnology will undoubtedly have great benefits in the long term in all sectors.

The growth in awareness of modern biotechnology parallels the serious worldwide changes in the economic climate arising from the escalation of oil prices since 1973. There is a growing realisation that fossil fuels and other non-renewable resources will one day be in limited supply. This will result in the requirement of cheaper and more secure energy sources and chemical feedstocks, which biotechnology could perhaps fulfil. Countries with climatic conditions that are suitable for rapid biomass production could well have major economic advantages over less climatically suitable parts of the world. In particular, the tropics must hold high future potential in this respect.

Another contributory factor regarding the growing interest in biotechnology has been the current recession in the western world, in particular the depression of the chemical and engineering sections, in part due to the increased energy costs. Biotechnology has been considered as one important means of restimulating the economy – whether on a local, regional, national or even global basis – using new biotechnological methods and new raw materials. In part, the industrial boom of the 1950s and 1960s was due to cheap oil, while the information technology advances in the 1970s and 1980s resulted from developments in microelectronics. It is quite feasible that the twenty-first century will increasingly be viewed as the era of biotechnology. There is undoubtedly a worldwide increase in molecular biological research, the formation of new biotechnological companies, and large investments by nations, companies and individuals, together with the rapid expansion of databases and information sources and, above all, extensive media coverage.

It is perhaps unfortunate that there has been an over-concentration on the new implications of biotechnology and less identification of the very large traditional biotechnological industrial bases which already function throughout the world and which contribute considerably to most nations' gross national profits. Indeed, many of the new innovations in biotechnology will not appear a priori as new products but rather as improvements to organisms and processes in long-established biotechnological industries, e.g. brewing and antibiotic production.

New applications are likely to be seen earliest in the area of health care and medicine, followed by agriculture and food technology. Exciting new medical treatments and drugs based on biotechnology are appearing with ever-increasing regularity. Prior to 1982, insulin for human diabetics was derived from beef and pork pancreases. The gene for human insulin was then isolated and cloned into microorganisms, which were then mass-produced by fermentation. This genetically engineered human insulin – identical to the natural human hormone – was the first commercial pharmaceutical product of recombinant DNA technology and now supplies millions of insulin users worldwide with a safe, reliable and unlimited source of this vital hormone. Biotechnology has also made it easier to detect and diagnose human, animal and plant diseases. In clinical diagnosis there are now hundreds of specialised kits available for simple home use or for complex laboratory procedures such as blood screening.

Biotechnology will be increasingly required to meet the global population's current and future needs for food products that are safe and nutritious while also ensuring a continuous improvement in the efficiency of food production. Acceptance of new food products produced using new biotechnology may be greater when consumers can readily see the benefits derived from novel

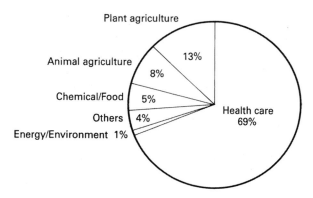

Fig. 1.2   Distribution of research and development funding in industrial biotechnology in the USA.

production methods. Biotechnology methods can now improve the nutrition, taste and appearance of plants and various food products, enhance resistance to specific viruses and insect pests, and produce safer herbicides. For food safety, new probes can rapidly detect and accurately identify specific microbial pathogens in food, e.g. *Salmonella, Listeria* and fungal toxins such as aflatoxin.

Increasingly, biotechnology will evolve as a powerful and versatile approach which can compete with chemical and physical techniques of reducing energy and material consumption and minimising the generation of waste and emissions. Biotechnology will be a valuable, indeed essential, contribution for achieving industrial sustainability in the future. There is an ever-increasing diversity and scale of raw material consumption and this means that it is becoming urgent to act to minimise the increasing pressures on the environment. Applications in chemical production, fuel and energy production, pollution control and resource recovery will possibly take longer to develop and will depend on changes in the relative economics of currently employed technologies.

The use of biotechnology with respect to the environment could have contrasting effects. On the one hand there would be many positive effects on environmental conservation, e.g. reduced contamination, improved recycling, and soil utilisation, etc., while on the other hand, the liberation of genetically modified organisms could generate some potential environmental risks, e.g. natural population displacements, ecological interactions and transfer of undesirable genetic characteristics to other species.

Figure 1.2 shows how the USA is currently applying R&D funding to industrial biotechnology.

Table 1.5. Some unique features of biotechnology companies

Technology-driven and multidisciplinary: product development can involve molecular biologists, clinical researchers, product sales force.

Must manage regulatory authorities, public perception; issues of health and safety; risk assessment.

Business climate characterised by rapid change and considerable risk – one biotechnology innovation may quickly supercede another.

Biotechnology business growth highly dependent on venture capital – usually needs exceptionally high level of funding before profit sales return.

Biotechnology-based industries will not be labour intensive, and although they will create valuable new employment, the need will be more for brains than muscle. Much of modern biotechnology has been developed and utilised by large companies and corporations. However, many small and medium-sized companies are realising that biotechnology is not a science of the future but provides real benefits to their industry today. In many industries traditional technology can produce compounds that cause environmental damage, whereas biotechnology methods can offer a 'green' alternative, promoting a positive public image and also avoiding new environmental penalties. Knowledge of biotechnology innovations must be translated through to all sectors of industry.

Many new, high-technology biotech companies have arisen from entrepreneurs from academia who are often dominant, charismatic individuals whose primary aim has been to develop a new technology. New biotechnology companies have certain features that are not often seen in others (Table 1.5). The position of new biotechnology at the interface between academia and industry creates a unique need for abstracting information from a wide range of sources; thus, companies spend large sums on information management.

Biotechnology is high technology *par excellence*. The most exciting and potentially profitable facets of new biotechnology in the next decade will involve research and development at the very frontiers of current knowledge and techniques.

In the late 1970s molecular biologists were putting forward vague promises about the wonders of this scientific discipline while the realising technologies were still being developed and were still requiring immense levels of research and product development fundings. Biotechnologists now make predictions with more confidence since many of the apparently insurmountable problems have been more easily overcome than had been predicted and many transitions from laboratory experiments to large-scale industrial processes have been achieved. Truly, new biotechnology has come of age.

For biotechnology to be commercially successful and exploited there is a need both to recruit a specialist workforce and also for the technology to be understood and applied by practitioners in a wide range of other areas, including law, patents, medicine, agriculture, engineering, etc. Higher education will supply the range of specialist disciplines encompassing biotechnology while some courses will endeavour to produce 'biotechnology' graduates who have covered many of the specialist areas at a less rigorous level than the 'pure degree' specialisation. Also, many already employed in biotechnology-based industries must regularly have means of updating or even retraining. To this end, there are now many books on specific aspects of biotechnology, together with software programs. The European-based BIOTOL (Biotechnology by Open Learning) has now produced a wide range of learning programmes. Such programmes are designed not only for the needs of students but also for company training activities and are written in a user-friendly style of good, open-learning materials. The currency of biotechnology throughout the world will be an educated, skilled workforce and ready access to the ever-widening knowledge and resource base. Science has defined the world in which we live, and biotechnology, in particular, will become an essential and accepted activity of our culture.

1.4   Biotechnology: a three-component central core

Many biotechnological processes may be considered as having a three-component central core, in which one part is concerned with obtaining the best biological catalyst for a specific function or process, the second part creates (by construction and technical operation) the best possible environment for the catalyst to perform, and the third part (downstream processing) is concerned with the separation and purification of an essential product or products from a fermentation process.

With regards to the first part of the biotechnology core, the most effective, stable and convenient form for the catalyst for a biotechnological process is a whole organism and it is for this reason that so much of biotechnology revolves around microbial processes. This does not exclude the use of higher organisms; in particular, plant and animal cell culture will play an increasingly important role in biotechnology.

Microorganisms can be viewed both as primary fixers of photosynthetic energy and as systems for bringing about chemical changes in almost all types of natural and synthetic organic molecules. Collectively, they have an immense gene pool which offers almost unlimited synthetic and degradative potential. Furthermore, microorganisms can possess extremely rapid growth rates far in excess of any of the higher organisms such as plants and animals. Thus immense quantities can be produced under the correct environmental conditions in short time periods.

The methodologies that are in general use enable the selection of improved microorganisms from the natural environmental pool, the modification of microorganisms by mutation and, more recently, the mobilisation of a spectacular array of new techniques, deriving from molecular biology, which may eventually permit the construction of microorganisms, plants and animals, with totally novel biochemical potentials (Chapter 3). These new techniques have largely arisen from fundamental achievements in molecular biology over the last two decades.

These manipulated and improved organisms must be maintained in substantially unchanged form and this involves another spectrum of techniques for the preservation of organisms, for retaining essential features during industrial processes and, above all, for retaining long-term vigour and viability. In many examples the catalyst is used in a separated and purified form, namely as enzymes, and a huge amount of information has been built up on the large-scale production, isolation and purification of individual enzymes and on their stabilization by artificial means (Chapter 5).

The second part of the core of biotechnology encompasses all aspects of the containment system or 'bioreactor' within which the catalysts must function (Chapter 4). Here the combined specialist knowledge of the bioscientist and bioprocess engineering will interact, providing the design and instrumentation for the maintenance and control of the physico-chemical environment, such as temperature, aeration, pH, etc., thus allowing the optimum expression of the biological properties of the catalyst. Having achieved the required endpoint of the biotechnological process within the bioreactor, e.g. biomass or biochemical product, in most cases it will be necessary to separate the organic products from the predominantly aqueous environment. This third aspect of biotechnology – 'downstream processing' – can be a technically difficult and expensive procedure, and is the least understood area of biotechnology. Downstream processing is primarily concerned with initial separation of the bioreactor broth or medium into a liquid phase and a solids phase, and subsequent concentration and purification of the product. Processing will usually involve more than one stage. Downstream processing costs (as approximate proportions of selling prices) of fermentation products vary considerably, e.g. with yeast biomass, penicillin G and certain enzymes,

Table 1.6. The main areas of application of biotechnology

Bioprocess technology
Historically, the most important area of biotechnology, namely brewing, antibiotics, mammalian cell culture, etc.; extensive development in progress with new products envisaged, namely polysaccharides, medically important drugs, solvents, protein-enhanced foods. Novel fermenter designs to optimize productivity.

Enzyme technology
Used for the catalysis of extremely specific chemical reactions; immobilization of enzymes; to create specific molecular converters (bioreactors). Products formed include L-amino acids, high fructose syrup, semi-synthetic penicillins, starch and cellulose hydrolysis, etc. Enzyme probes for bioassays.

Waste technology
Long historical importance but more emphasis now being made to couple these processes with the conservation and recycling of resources; foods and fertilizers, biological fuels.

Environmental technology
Great scope exists for the application of biotechnological concepts for solving many environmental problems – pollution control, removing toxic wastes; recovery of metals from mining wastes and low-grade ores.

Renewable resources technology
The use of renewable energy sources, in particular lignocellulose, to generate new sources of chemical raw materials and energy – ethanol, methane and hydrogen. Total utilisation of plant and animal material. Clean technology, sustainable technology.

Plant and animal agriculture
Genetically engineered plants for improved nutrition, disease resistance, keeping quality; improved yields and stress tolerance will become increasingly commercially available. Improved productivity, etc., for animal farming. Improved food quality, flavour, taste and microbial safety.

Health care
New drugs and better treatment for delivering medicines to diseased parts. Improved disease diagnosis, understanding of the human genome – genomics and proteomics, information technology.

processing costs as percentages of selling prices are 20%, 20–30% and 60–70% respectively.

Successful involvement in a biotechnological process must draw heavily upon more than one of the input disciplines. The main areas of application of biotechnology are shown in Table 1.6 while Fig. 1.3 attempts to show how

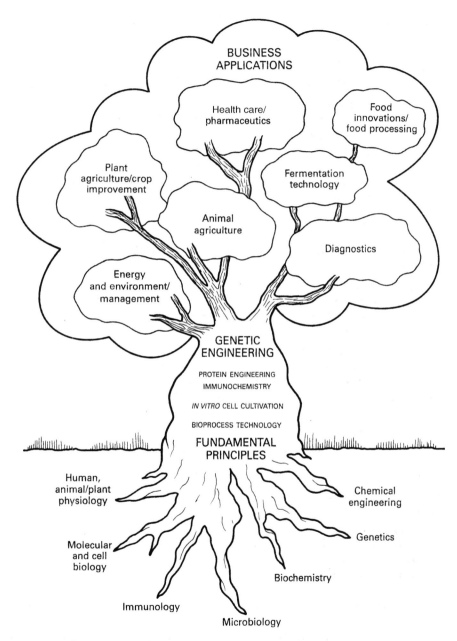

Fig. 1.3 The biotechnology tree.

the many disciplines are input into the biotechnological processes together with the differing enabling technologies.

Biotechnology will continue to create exciting new opportunities for commercial development and profits in a wide range of industrial sectors, including health care and medicine, agriculture and forestry, fine and bulk chemicals production, food technology, fuel and energy production, pollution control and resource recovery. Biotechnology offers a great deal of hope for solving many of the problems the world faces!

1.5   Product safety

In biotechnology, governmental regulations will represent a critical determinant on the time and total costs in bringing a product to market. Regulatory agencies can act as 'gate-keepers' for the development and availability of new biotechnology products but can also erect considerable barriers to industrial development. In practice, such barriers come from the costs of testing products to meet regulatory standards, possible delays and uncertainties in regulatory approval, and even outright disapproval of new products on grounds of safety. The very considerable costs that may be required to ensure product safety can often discourage new research or curtail product development if a future new product is not likely to have a high financial market return. Concern has been expressed in the USA that over-zealous and perhaps unrealistic regulatory requirements are damaging the future industrial development of some areas of biotechnology and, consequently, are systematically de-escalating their regulatory requirements. The use of recombinant DNA technology has created the greatest areas of possible safety concern (Chapters 13, 14). Public attitudes to biotechnology are most often related to matters of perceived or imaginary dangers in the techniques of genetic manipulation.

1.6   Public perception of biotechnology

While biotechnology presents enormous potential for health care and the production, processing and quality of foods by genetic engineering of crops, fertilisers, pesticides, vaccines and various animal and fish species, the implications of these new biotechnological processes go well beyond the technical benefits offered. The implementation of the new techniques will be dependent upon their acceptance by consumers (Chapter 14). As stated in the ACOST (Advisory Committee on Science and Technology), report *Developments in*

Biotechnology': 'Public perception of biotechnology will have a major influence on the rate and direction of developments and there is growing concern about genetically modified products. Associated with genetic manipulation are diverse questions of safety, ethics and welfare.'

Public debate is essential for new biotechnology to grow up and undoubtedly for the foreseeable future biotechnology will be under scrutiny. Public understanding of these new technologies could well hasten public acceptance. However, the low level of scientific literacy (e.g. in the USA, where only 7% are scientifically literate) does mean that most of the public will not be able to draw informed conclusions about important biotechnology issues. Consequently, it is conceivable (and indeed occurring) for a small number of activists to argue the case against genetic engineering in such emotive and ill-reasoned ways that the public and the politicians are misled. The biotechnology community needs to sit up and take notice of, and work with, the public. People influence decision making by governments through the ballot box or through the presence of public opinion.

Ultimately the benefits of biotechnology will speak for themselves, as will be seen in the following chapters.

1.7 Biotechnology and the developing world

Successful agriculture holds the answer to the poverty gap between the rich and poor nations. In the developed world agricultural sciences are well developed, producing an abundance of high-quality products. Agricultural biotechnology (Chapter 10) will further improve quality, variety and yield. Will these new plant species, improved by genetic engineering, find their way to the developing countries, ensuring higher productivity, greater resistance to disease and more marketability? It is not yet clear what will happen other than that the affluent nations will become increasingly well endowed with an abundance of food. Worldwide, there will be enough food for all but will it always continue to be disproportionately distributed? Biotechnology developments need high inputs of finance and a skilled workforce – both of which are in short supply in most developing nations. Sadly, there is a growing gap between biotechnology in highly industrialised countries and the biotechnology-based needs of developing countries.

While many developing nations have successfully collaborated in the past with western biotechnology companies, it is salutary to note that between 1986 and 1991 the percentage of arrangements implemented by US biotechnology companies with developing countries dropped from 20% to 3%! The ability of developing nations to avail themselves of the many promises of new biotechnology will, to a large extent, depend on their capacity to integrate modern developments of biotechnology within their own research and innovation systems, in accordance with their own needs and priorities.

In the following chapters some of the most important areas of biotechnology are considered with a view to achieving a broad overall understanding of the existing achievements and future aims of this new area of technology. However, it must be appreciated that biotechnological development will not only depend on scientific and technological advances, but will also be subject to considerable political, economic and, above all, public acceptance. Finally, it has been said that most scientific disciplines pass through 'golden ages' when new approaches open the door to rapid and fundamental expansion. Biotechnology is just now entering this golden period. A spectacular future lies ahead.

2

Substrates for biotechnology

2.1 A biomass strategy

It has been estimated that the annual net yield of plant biomass arising from photosynthesis is at least 120 billion tonnes of dry matter on land and about 50 billion tonnes from the world's oceans. Of the land-produced biomass, approximately 50% occurs in the complex form of lignocellulose.

The highest proportion of land-based biomass (44%) is produced as forest (Table 2.1). It is surprising to note that while agricultural crops account for only 6% of the primary photosynthetic productivity, from this amount is derived a major portion of food for humans and animals as well as many essential structural materials, textiles and paper products (Table 2.2). Many traditional agricultural products may well be further exploited with the increasing awareness of biotechnology. In particular, new technological approaches will undoubtedly be able to utilise the large volume of waste material from conventional food processing that presently finds little use.

Biomass agriculture, aquaculture and forestry may hold great economic potential for many national economies, particularly in tropical and subtropical regions (Fig. 2.1). Indeed, the development of biotechnological processes in developing areas where plant growth excels could well bring about a change in the balance of economic power.

It should be noted that the non-renewable energy and petrochemical feedstocks on which modern society is so dependent, namely oil, gas and coal, were derived from ancient types of biomass. Modern industrialised nations have come to rely heavily on fossil reserves for both energy and as feedstocks for a wide range of production processes. In little over a century the industrialised

Table 2.1. Breakdown of world primary productivity

Category	Net productivity (% of total)
Forests and woodlands	44.3
Grassland	9.7
Cultivated land	5.9
Desert and semi-desert	1.5
Freshwater	3.2
Oceans	35.4

Table 2.2. Approximate annual world production of some agricultural and forestry products

Sector	Product	Tonnes	Value ($US billion)
Food and feed	Cereals (including milled rice)	1.8 billion	±250
	Sugar (cane and beet)	120 million	
	Fish	85 million	17
	Crude starch	1.0 billion	
	Refined starch	20 million	
Materials	Potential wood	13 billion	
	Harvested wood	1.6 billion	
	Fuel wood		100
	Saw wood		60
	Panels		35
	Paper		110
Chemicals	Oils and fats	70 million	
	Soybean oil	17 million	8
	Palm oil	10 million	3
	Sunflower oil	8 million	4
	Rape seed oil	8 million	3
	Starch	2 million	
	Natural pulses	4 million	4
Other	Cut flowers and bulbs		10
	Tobacco	4 million	15

From Organisation for Economic Cooperation and Development (1992).

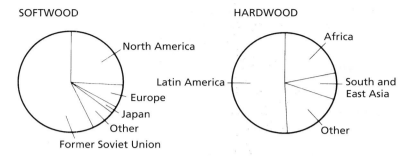

Fig. 2.1   The distribution of world forestry resources.

world has drawn heavily on fossil fuels that took millions of years to form beneath the beds of the oceans or in the depths of the earth. Furthermore, it is a very unequal pattern of usage. At present, the USA with 6% and western Europe with 8% of the world's population use 35% and 25% respectively of the world's oil and gas productions.

While coal stocks may last for many hundreds of years, this is not true for oil and gas, and at current usage levels the world's known available sources of oil and gas will have been almost fully exploited by the end of this century. The answer to these problems must be the use of photosynthetically derived biomass for energy and industrial feedstocks. Currently more than ten times more energy is generated annually by photosynthesis than is consumed by mankind. At present, large-scale exploitation of biomass for fuel and chemical feedstocks is restricted by the low cost of fossil alternatives, the heterogeneous nature of biomass sources and the diffuse distribution.

The use of biomass directly as a source of energy has long been practised in the less industrialised nations such as Latin America, China, India and Africa. In developed nations, biomass derived from agriculture and forestry has largely been directed to industrial and food uses (Table 2.3).

At present, biomass is used to derive many products of industrial and commercial importance (Table 2.3); those products that involve biotechnology will be highlighted and expanded on in subsequent chapters.

2.2   Natural raw materials

Natural raw materials originate mostly from agriculture and forestry. These are mainly carbohydrates of varying chemical complexity and include sugar, starch, cellulose, hemicellulose and lignin. The wide range of by-products

Table 2.3. Important products derived from biomass

Sector	Derived product
Fuels	Methane (biogas) – especially in the developing world
	Pyrolysis products (gas, charcoal)
	Ethanol (via cane juice and cellulose fermentation)
	Oils (from hydrogenation)
	Direct combustion of waste biomass
Feedstocks	Ethanol (potential feedstock for industry)
	Synthesis gas (from chemical gasification)
Fertilisers	Compost
	Sludge
Feeds	Direct feed supplements
	Single cell proteins

obtained from raw materials and of use in biotechnological processes is shown in Table 2.4.

Sugar-bearing raw materials such as sugar beet, sugar cane and sugar millet are the most suitable and available to serve as feedstocks for biotechnological processing. As traditional uses of sugar are replaced by more efficient alternatives, the sugar surplus on the commodity market will give further incentive to develop new uses. Many tropical economies would collapse if the market for sugar were to be removed. Already cane sugar serves as the substrate for the Brazilian gasohol programme, and many other nations are rapidly seeing the immense potential of these new technologies.

Starch-bearing agricultural products include various types of grain, such as maize, rice and wheat, together with potatoes and other root crops, such as sweet potato and cassava. A slight disadvantage of starch is that it must usually be degraded to monosaccharides or oligosaccharides by digestion or hydrolysis before fermentation. However, many biotechnological processes using starch are being developed, including fuel production.

There can be little doubt that cellulose – both from agriculture and from forestry sources – must contribute a major source of feedstock for biotechnological processes such as the production of fuels and chemicals. However, cellulose is a very complex chemical and invariably occurs in nature in close association with lignin. The ability of lignocellulose complexes to withstand the biodegradative forces of nature is witnessed by the longevity of trees, which are mainly composed of lignocellulose.

Lignocellulose is the most abundant and renewable natural resource available to man throughout the world. However, massive technological difficulties

Table 2.4. A range of by-products that could be used as substrates in biotechnology

By-product		
Agriculture	Forestry	Industry
Straw	Wood waste hydrolysate	Molasses
Bagasse	Sulphite pulp liquor	Distillery wastes
Maize cobs	Bark, sawdust, branches	Whey
Coffee, cocoa and coconut hulls	Paper and cellulose Fibres	Industrial waste water from food industries (olive, palm oil, potato, date, citrus, cassava)
Fruit peels and leaves		Wash waters (dairy, canning, confectionery, bakery, soft
Tea wastes		drinks, sizing, malting, corn steep)
Oilseed cakes		Fishery effluent and wastes
Cotton wastes		Meat by-products
Bran		Municipal garbage
Pulp (tomato, coffee, banana, pineapple, citrus, olive)		Sewage Abattoir wastes
Animal wastes		

must be overcome before economic use may be made of this plentiful compound. At present, expensive energy-demanding pre-treatment processes are required to open up this complex structure to wide microbial degradation. Pure cellulose can be degraded by chemical or enzymatic hydrolysis to soluble sugars, which can be fermented to form ethanol, butanol, acetone, single cell protein, methane and many other products. Exciting advances are being made in laboratories throughout the world and it is only a matter of time before these difficulties are overcome. It has been realistically calculated that approximately 3.3×10^{14} kg of CO_2 per year are fixed on the surface of the earth and that approximately 6% of this, i.e. 22 billion tonnes per year, will be cellulose. On a worldwide basis, land plants produce 24 tonnes of cellulose per person per year. Time will surely show that lignocellulose will be the most useful carbon source for biotechnological developments.

2.3   Availability of by-products

While biotechnological processes will use many agricultural products such as sugars, starches, oils, etc., as substrates, the vast array of waste products derived from agriculture, and currently not creatively used, will undoubtedly be subjected to detailed examination and future utilisation. Agricultural and forestry wastes come in many diverse types: cereal straws, corn husks and cobs, soy wastes, coconut shells, rice husks, coffee bean husks, wheat bran, sugar cane bagasse and forestry wastes, including trimmings, sawdust, bark, etc. (Table 2.4). Only a modest fraction of these wastes are utilised on a large scale owing primarily to economic and logistical factors.

A primary objective of biotechnology is to improve the management and utilisation of the vast volumes of agricultural, industrial and domestic waste organic materials to be found throughout the world. The biotechnological utilisation of these wastes will eliminate a source of pollution, in particular water pollution, and convert some of these wastes into useful by-products.

Not all of these processes will involve biosystems. In particular, the processes of reverse osmosis and ultrafiltration are finding increasing uses. Reverse osmosis is a method of concentrating liquid solutions in which a porous membrane allows water to pass through but not the salts dissolved in it. Ultrafiltration is a method of separating the high- and low-molecular-weight compounds in a liquid by allowing the liquid and low-molecular-weight compounds to pass through while holding back the high-molecular-weight compounds and suspended solids. Some current applications of these technologies include concentration of dilute factory effluents, concentration of dilute food products, sterilisation of water, purification of brackish water, and separation of edible solids from dilute effluents.

Waste materials are frequently important for economic and environmental reasons. For example, many by-products of the food industry are of low economic value and are often discharged into waterways, creating serious environmental pollution problems. An attractive feature of carbohydrate waste as a raw material is that, if its low cost can be coupled with suitable low handling costs, an economic process may be obtained. Furthermore, the worldwide trend towards stricter effluent control measures, or parallel increase in effluent disposal charges, can lead to the concept of waste as a 'negative cost' raw material. However, the composition or dilution of the waste may be so dispersed that transport to a production centre may be prohibitive. On these occasions biotechnology may only serve to reduce a pollution hazard.

Each waste material must be assessed for its suitability for biotechnological processing. Only when a waste is available in large quantities, and preferably over a prolonged period of time, can a suitable method of utilisation be considered (Table 2.5).

Table 2.5. Biotechnological strategies for the utilisation of suitable organic waste materials

(1) Upgrading the food waste quality to make it suitable for human consumption
(2) Feeding the food waste directly, or after processing, to poultry, pigs, fish or other single-stomach animals which can utilise it directly
(3) Feeding the food waste to cattle or other ruminants if unsuitable for single-stomach animals because of high fibre content, toxins or other reasons
(4) Production of biogas (methane) and other fermentation products if unsuitable for feeding without expensive pre-treatments
(5) Selective other purposes such as direct use as fuel, building materials, chemical extraction, etc.

Two widely occurring wastes which already find considerable fermentation uses are molasses and whey. Molasses is a by-product of the sugar industry and has a sugar content of approximately 50%. Molasses is widely used as a fermentation feedstock for the production of antibiotics, organic acids and commercial yeasts for baking, and is directly used in animal feeding. Whey, obtained during the production of cheese, could also become a major fermentation feedstock.

More complex wastes such as straw and bagasse are widely available and will be increasingly used as improved processes for lignocellulose breakdown become available (Table 2.6). Wood wastes will include low-grade wood, bark and sawdust, as well as waste liquors such as sulphite waste liquor from pulp production, which already finds considerable biotechnological processing in Europe and former Communist-bloc countries (Chapter 7).

The largest proportion of total volume of waste matter is from animal rearing (faeces, urine), then agricultural wastes, then wastes from food industries, and finally domestic wastes. The disposal of many waste materials, particularly animal wastes, is no problem in traditional agriculture and is particularly well exemplified in China where recycling by composting has long been practised. However, where intensive animal rearing is undertaken, serious pollution problems do arise.

2.4   Chemical and petrochemical feedstocks

With the development of commercial processes for the production of single cell protein (SCP) and other organic products, a number of chemical and petrochemical feedstocks have become particularly important for fermentation

Table 2.6. Pre-treatments required before substrates are suitable for fermentation

Substrate	Pre-treatment
Sugary materials	
Sugar cane, beet, molasses, fruit juices, whey	Minimal requirements of dilution and sterilisation.
Starchy materials	
Cereals, rice, vegetables, process liquid wastes	Some measure of hydrolysis by acid or enzymes. Initial separation of non-starch components may be required.
Lignocellulosic materials	
Corn cobs, oat hulls, straw, bagasse, wood wastes, sulphite liquor, paper wastes	Normally requires complex pre-treatment involving reduction in particle size followed by various chemical or enzymic hydrolyses. Energy intensive and costly.

processes since these materials have the advantage of being available in large quantities and in the same quality in most parts of the world. Thus, natural gas or methane and gas oil have been preferred as raw material because of their easy processing and universal availability. Main commercial interest has been concerned with *n*-paraffins, methanol and ethanol. Their involvement in various aspects of biotechnology, particularly in SCP production, will be considered later.

Future biotechnological processes will increasingly make use of organic materials which are renewable in nature or which occur as low-value wastes which may presently cause environmental pollution. Table 2.7 summarises the many technical considerations that must be made when approaching the utilisation of waste materials. Some processes may also more economically utilise specific fractions of fossil fuels as feedstocks for biotechnological processes.

2.5 Raw materials and the future of biotechnology

It is now clear that the future development of large-scale biotechnological processes is inseparable from the supply and cost of raw materials. During the early and middle parts of the last century, the availability of cheap oil led to an explosive development of the petrochemical industry, and many products formally derived from the fermentation ability of microorganisms

Table 2.7. Technical considerations for the utilisation of waste materials

Consideration	Related factor
Biological availability	*Low* (cellulosics) *Moderate* (starch, lactose) *High* (molasses, pulping sugars)
Concentration	*Solid* (milling residues, garbage) *Concentrated* (molasses) *Weak* (lactose, pulping sugars) *Very dilute* (process and plant wash liquors)
Quality	*Clean* (molasses, lactose) *Moderate* (straw) *Dirty* (garbage, feedlot waste)
Location	*Collected* (large installation, small centres) *Collected specialised* (olive, palm oil, date, rubber, fruit, vegetables) *Dispersed* (straw, forestry)
Seasonal availability	*Prolonged* (palm oil, lactose) *Very short* (vegetable cannery waste)
Alternative uses	*Some* (straw) *None* (garbage) *Negative* (costly effluents)
Local technology potential	*High* (USA) *Middle* (Brazil) *Low* (Malaysia)

were superseded by the cheaper and more efficient chemical methods. However, escalating oil prices in the 1970s created profound reappraisals of these processes and, as the price of crude oil approached that of some major cereal products (Fig. 2.2), there was a reawakening of interest in many fermentation processes for the production of ethanol and related products. However, the decrease in oil prices in 1986 again widened the gap and left uncertainty in the minds of industrial planners.

The most important criteria in determining the selection of a raw material for a biotechnological process will include price, availability, composition and form and oxidation state of the carbon source. Table 2.8 provides interesting details on the mid-1984 prices of existing and potential raw materials of biotechnological interest. At present, the most widely used and of most commercial value are corn starch, methanol, molasses and raw sugar.

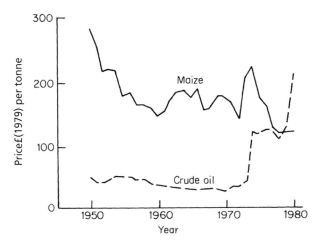

Fig. 2.2 Prices of maize and crude oil, 1950–1980 (from King, 1982).

There is little doubt that cereal crops, particularly maize, rice and wheat, will be the main short- and medium-term raw materials for biotechnological processes. Furthermore, it is believed that this can be achieved without seriously disturbing human and animal food supplies. Throughout the world there is an uneven distribution of cereal production capacity and demand. Overproduction of cereals occurs mostly where extensive biotechnological processes are in practice. Areas of poor cereal production will undoubtedly benefit from the developments in agricultural biotechnology that are now at an early but highly optimistic stage.

Although much attention has been given to the uses of wastes in biotechnology, they are many major obstacles to be overcome. For instance, availability of agricultural wastes is seasonal and geographic availability problematic; they are also often dilute and may contain toxic wastes. However, their build-up in the environment can present serious pollution problems and therefore their utilisation in biotechnological processes, albeit at little economic gain, can have overall community value.

Although in the long term biotechnology must seek to utilise the components of cellulose and lignocelluloses as fuels or feedstocks, the technological difficulties are still considerable. The chemical complexity of these molecules is legendary and it is proving more difficult than had been expected to economically break them down to usable primary molecules.

Biotechnology will have profound effects on agriculture and forestry by enabling production costs to be decreased, quality and consistency of products to be increased, and novel products generated.

Table 2.8. Prices of available raw materials for biotechnological processes

Substrate	Mid-1984 US price ($ per tonne)	Carbon content (g per mol C per mol substrate)	Carbon content relative to glucose (%)	Corrected price relative to glucose ($ per tonne)[a]
Corn starch	70–100[b]	0.44	100	64–91
Glucose	290[c]	0.4	100	290
Sucrose – raw	140[d]	0.42	105	133
Sucrose – refined	660[e]	0.42	105	140
Molasses	79	0.2[f]	50	140
Acetic acid	550	0.4	100	550
Ethanol	560	0.52	130	430
Methane	n.a.	0.75	188	—
Corn oil (crude)	330	0.8	200	165
Palm oil	600	0.8	200	300
n-alkanes (n-hexadecane)	n.a.	0.87	218	—

n.a. Not available.
[a] Assumes equivalent conversion efficiencies can be obtained.
[b] Approximate guessed price in a wet-milling operation.
[c] Glucose syrups on a dry-weight basis.
[d] Daily spot price.
[e] US price fixed by government tariffs.
[f] On the basis of molasses being 48% by weight fermentable sugars.
From Hacking (1986).

Wood is extensively harvested to provide fuel and materials for construction and to supply pulp for paper manufacture. Supplies throughout the world are rapidly decreasing, due to extensive examples of deforestation: deforestation can often then be followed by desertification and soil erosion. Selective breeding programmes are now producing 'elite' fast-growing hardwood trees, such as eucalyptus and acacia, derived from genetic manipulation programmes coupled with new methods of macro- and micropropagation (Chapter 10). Such fast-growing trees could even be used for electricity generation, producing less net overall CO_2 than the use of fossil fuels and so minimising any potential 'greenhouse' effect.

There may also be an increased non-food use of many agriculturally derived substances such as sugars, starches, oils and fats. Biotechnology will significantly aid their overall production by improved plant growth, influence biosynthetic pathways to change production, change the chemical structure of molecules, and improve processing by enzyme technology. The ability of biotechnology to improve disease resistance and quality composition and, in some cases, to grow crops in marginal lands could surely lead to higher yields of products, and in developing economies this could have profound beneficial effects. Supplies in excess of food needs could allow new industries to develop and reduce poverty.

Cotton is a major agricultural crop in many developing nations and is a major natural textile fibre, with world production exceeding that of synthetic textile fibres. It is not well recognised that cotton accounts for about 10% of the world's annual use of agrochemicals, mainly insecticides. Development of disease-resistant cotton plants by new molecular methods could have major economical and environmental impact. Major yield increases would have considerable benefits to the producing nations.

How successful will biomass be as a crucial raw material for biotechnology? An OECD report (1992) set out the factors which will determine the competitiveness of natural (biomass) and synthetic (fossil biomass) derived products:

(1) the relative price of the basic raw materials.
(2) quality, variability, regularity of supply and safety of the raw materials.
(3) relative costs of chemical base material conversion compared to conversion of agricultural products.
(4) premium accorded by the market to 'natural' as compared to synthetic products and increasing requirement for products to be biodegradable.

3

Genetics and biotechnology

3.1   Introduction

In essence, all properties of organisms depend on the sum of their genes. There are two broad categories of genes: structural and regulatory. *Structural genes* encode for amino acid sequences of proteins which, as enzymes, determine the biochemical capabilities of the organism by catalysing particular synthetic or catabolic reactions or, alternatively, play more static roles as components of cellular structures. In contrast, the *regulatory genes* control the expression of the structural genes by determining the rate of production of their protein products in response to intra- or extracellular signals. The derivation of these principles has been achieved using well- known genetic techniques which will not be considered further here.

The seminal studies of Watson and Crick and others in the early 1950s led to the construction of the double-helix model depicting the molecular structure of DNA and subsequent hypotheses on its implications for the understanding of gene replication. Since then there has been a spectacular unravelling of the complex interactions required to express the coded chemical information of the DNA molecule into cellular and organismal expression. Changes in the DNA molecule making up the genetic complement of an organism is the means by which organisms evolve and adapt themselves to new environments. In nature, changes in the DNA of an organism can occur in two ways:

(1) By *mutation*, which is a chemical deletion or addition of one or more of the chemical parts of the DNA molecule.

(2) By the interchange of genetic information or DNA between like organisms normally by *sexual reproduction* and by *horizontal transfer* in bacteria. In eukaryotes, sexual reproduction is achieved by a process of conjugation in which there is a donor, called 'male', and a recipient, called 'female'. Often, these are determined physiologically and not morphologically. Bacterial conjugation involves the transfer of DNA from a donor to a recipient cell. The transferred DNA (normally plasmid DNA) is always in a single-stranded form and the complementary strand is synthesised in the recipient. *Transduction* is the transfer of DNA mediated by a bacterial virus (*bacteriophage* or *phage*), and cells that have received transducing DNA are referred to as '*transductants*'. *Transformation* involves the uptake of isolated DNA, or DNA present in the organism's environment, into a recipient cell which is then referred to as a '*transformant*'. Genetic transfer by this way in bacteria is a natural characteristic of a wide variety of bacterial genera such a *Campylobacter, Neisseria* and *Streptomyces*. Strains of bacteria that are not naturally transformable can be induced to take up isolated DNA by chemical treatment or by *electroporation*.

Classical genetics was, until recently, the only way in which heredity could be studied and manipulated. However, in recent years, new techniques have permitted unprecedented alterations in the genetic make-up of organisms, even allowing exchange in the laboratory of DNA between unlike organisms.

The manipulation of the genetic material in organisms can now be achieved in three clearly definable ways: organismal, cellular and molecular.

Organismal manipulation

Genetic manipulation of whole organisms has been happening naturally by sexual reproduction since the beginning of time. The evolutionary progress of almost all living creatures has involved active interaction between their genomes and the environment. Active control of sexual reproduction has been practised in agriculture for decades – even centuries. In more recent times it has been used with several industrial microorganisms, e.g. yeasts. It involves selection, mutation, sexual crosses, hybridisation, etc. However, it is a very random process and can take a long time to achieve desired results – if at all in some cases. In agriculture, the benefits have been immense with much improved plants and animals, while in the biotechnological industries there has been greatly improved productivity, e.g. antibiotics and enzymes.

Cellular manipulation

Cellular manipulations of DNA have been used for over two decades, and involve either cell fusion or the culture of cells and the regeneration of whole plants from these cells (Chapter 10). This is a semi-random or directed process in contrast to organismal manipulations, and the changes can be more readily identified. Successful biotechnological examples of these methods include monoclonal antibodies and the cloning of many important plant species.

Molecular manipulation

Molecular manipulations of DNA and RNA first occurred over two decades ago and heralded a new era of genetic manipulations enabling – for the first time in biological history – a directed control of the changes. This is the much publicised area of *genetic engineering* or *recombinant DNA technology*, which is now bringing dramatic changes to biotechnology. In these techniques the experimenter is able to know much more about the genetic changes being made. It is now possible to add or delete parts of the DNA molecule with a high degree of precision, and the product can be easily identified. Current industrial ventures are concerned with the production of new types of organism and numerous compounds ranging from pharmaceuticals to commodity chemicals, and are discussed in more detail in later chapters.

3.2   Industrial genetics

Biotechnology has so far been considered as an interplay between two components, one of which is the selection of the best biocatalyst for a particular process, while the other is the construction and operation of the best environment for the catalyst to achieve optimum operation.

The most effective, stable and convenient form for the biocatalyst is a whole organism; in most cases it is some type of microbe, e.g. a bacterium, yeast or mould, although mammalian cell cultures and (to a lesser extent) plant cell cultures are finding ever-increasing uses in biotechnology.

Most microorganisms used in current biotechnological processes were originally isolated from the natural environment, and have subsequently been modified by the industrial geneticist into superior organisms for specific productivity. The success of strain selection and improvement programmes practised by all biologically based industries (e.g. brewing, antibiotics, etc.) is a direct result of the close cooperation between the technologist and the geneticist. In the future, this relationship will be even more necessary in formulating the specific physiological and biochemical characteristics that are sought in new organisms in order to give the fullest range of biological activities to biotechnology.

In biotechnological processes, the aim is primarily to optimise the particular characteristics sought in an organism, e.g. specific enzyme production or by-product formation. Genetic modification to improve productivity has been widely practised. The task of improving yields of some primary metabolites and macromolecules (e.g. enzymes) is simpler than trying to improve the yields of complex products such as antibiotics. Advances have been achieved in this area by using *screening* and *selection* techniques to obtain better organisms. In a selection system, all rare or novel strains grow while the rest do not; in a screening system, all strains grow but certain strains or cultures are chosen because they show the desired qualities required by the industry in question.

In most industrial genetics the basis for changing the organism's genome has been by mutation using X-rays and mutagenic chemicals. However, such methods normally lead only to the loss of undesired characters or increased production due to loss of control functions. It has rarely led to the appearance of a new function or property. Thus, an organism with a desired feature will be selected from the natural environment, propagated and subjected to a mutational programme, then screened to select the best progeny.

Unfortunately, many of the microorganisms that have gained industrial importance do not have a clearly defined sexual cycle. In particular, this has been the case in antibiotic-producing microorganisms; this has meant that the only way to change the genome, with a view to enhancing productivity, has been to indulge in massive mutational programmes followed by screening and selection to detect the new variants that might arise.

Once a high-producing strain has been found, great care is required in maintaining the strain. Undesired spontaneous mutations can sometimes occur at a high rate, giving rise to degeneration of the strain's industrial importance. Strain instability is a constant problem in industrial utilisation of microorganisms. Industry has always placed great emphasis on strain viability and productivity potential of the preserved biological material. Most industrially important microorganisms can be stored for long periods, for example in liquid nitrogen, by lyophilisation (freeze-drying) or under oil, and still retain their desired biological properties.

However, despite elaborate preservation and propagation methods, a strain has generally to be grown in a large-production bioreactor in which the chances of genetic changes through spontaneous mutation and selection are very high.

The chance of a high rate of spontaneous mutation is probably greater when the industrial strains in use have resulted from many years of mutagen treatment. Great secrecy surrounds the use of industrial microorganisms and immense care is taken to ensure that they do not unwittingly pass to outside agencies (Section 12.2).

There is now a growing movement away from the extreme empiricism that characterised the early days of the fermentation industries. Fundamental studies of the genetics of microorganisms now provide a background of knowledge for the experimental solution of industrial problems and increasingly contribute to progress in industrial strain selection.

In recent years, industrial genetics has come to depend increasingly on two new ways of manipulating DNA: – (1) protoplast and cell fusion, and (2) recombinant DNA technology (genetic engineering). These are now important additions to the technical repertoire of the geneticists involved with biotechnological industries. A brief examination of these techniques will attempt to show their increasingly indispensable relevance to modern biotechnology.

3.3   Protoplast and cell-fusion technologies

Plants and most microbial cells are characterised by a distinct outer wall or exoskeleton which gives the shape characteristic to the cell or organism. Immediately within the cell wall is the living membrane, or plasma membrane, retaining all the cellular components such as nuclei, mitochondria, vesicles, etc. For some years now it has been possible, using special techniques (in particular, hydrolytic enzymes), to remove the cell wall, releasing spherical membrane-bound structures known as *protoplasts*. These protoplasts are extremely fragile but can be maintained in isolation for variable periods of time. Isolated protoplasts cannot propagate themselves as such, requiring first the regeneration of a cell wall before regaining reproductive capacity.

In practice, it is the cell wall which largely hinders the sexual conjugation of unlike organisms. Only with completely sexually compatible strains does the wall degenerate, allowing protoplasmic interchange. Thus natural sexual mating barriers in microorganisms may, in part, be due to cell-wall limitations, and by removing this cell wall, the likelihood of cellular fusions may increase.

Protoplasts can be obtained routinely from many plant species, bacteria, yeasts and filamentous fungi. Protoplasts from different strains can sometimes be persuaded to fuse and so overcome the natural sexual mating barriers. However, the range of protoplast fusions is severely limited by the need for

DNA compatibility between the strains concerned. Fusion of protoplasts can be enhanced by treatment with the chemical polyethylene glycol, which, under optimum conditions, can lead to extremely high frequencies of recombinant formation which can be increased still further by ultraviolet irradiation of the parental protoplast preparations. Protoplast fusion can also occur with human or animal cell types.

Protoplast fusion has obvious empirical applications in yield improvement of antibiotics by combining yield-enhancing mutations from different strains or even species. Protoplasts will also be an important part of genetic engineering, in facilitating recombinant DNA transfer. Fusion may provide a method of re-assorting whole groups of genes between different strains of macro- and microorganisms.

One of the most exciting and commercially rewarding areas of biotechnology involves a form of mammalian cell fusion leading to the formation of monoclonal antibodies. It has long been recognised that certain cells (β-lymphocytes) within the body of vertebrates have the ability to secrete antibodies which can inactivate contaminating or foreign molecules (the antigen) within the animal system. The antibody has a Y-shaped molecular structure and uses one part of this structure to bind the invading antigen and the other part to trigger the body's response to eliminate the antigen/antibody complex. It has been calculated that a mammalian species can generate up to 100 million different antibodies, thereby ensuring that most invading foreign antigens will be bound by some antibody. Antibodies have high binding affinities and specificity against the chosen antigen. For the mammalian system it is the major defence against disease-causing organisms and other toxic molecules.

Attempts to cultivate the antibody-producing cells in artificial media have generally proved unsuccessful, with the cells either dying or ceasing to produce the antibodies. It is now known that individual β-lymphocyte cells produce single-antibody types. However, in 1975, Georges Köhler and Cesar Milstein successfully demonstrated the production of pure or *monoclonal antibodies* from the fusion product (*hybridoma*) of β-lymphocytes (antibody-producing cells) and myeloma tumour cells. In 1984, they were awarded the Nobel Prize for this outstanding scientific achievement. The commercial importance of their scientific findings can be judged from the estimate that, in the late 1990s, the value of therapeutic antibodies alone was $6 billion.

The monoclonal-antibody technique changes antibody-secreting cells (with limited life span) into cells that are capable of continuous growth (immortalisation) while maintaining their specific antibody-secreting potential. This immortalisation is achieved by a fusion technique, whereby β-lymphocyte cells are fused to 'immortal' cancer or myeloma cells in a one-to-one ratio, forming hybrids or hybridomas that are capable of continuous growth and

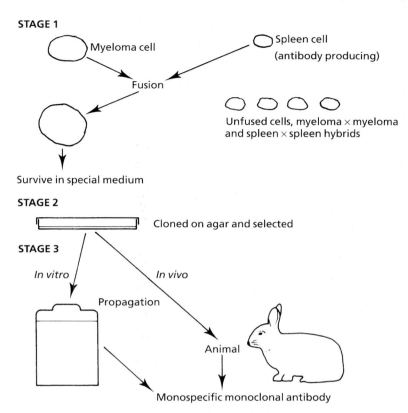

Fig. 3.1 The formation of antibody-producing hybridomas by fusion techniques. Stage 1: myeloma cells and antibody-producing cells (derived from immunised animal or man) are incubated in a special medium containing polyethylene glycol, which enhances fusion. Stage 2: the myeloma spleen hybridoma cells are selected out and cultured in closed agar dishes. Stage 3: the specific antibody-producing hybridoma is selected and propagated in culture vessels (*in vitro*) or in animal (*in vivo*) and monoclonal antibodies are harvested.

antibody secretion in culture. Single hybrid cells can then be selected and grown as clones or pure cultures of the hybridomas. Such cells continue to secrete antibody, and the antibody is of one particular specificity, as opposed to the mixture of antibodies that occurs in an animal's bloodstream after conventional methods of immunisation.

Monoclonal antibody formation is performed by injecting a mouse or rabbit with the antigen, later removing the spleen, and then allowing fusion of individual spleen cells with individual myeloma cells. Approximately 1% of the spleen cells are antibody-secreting cells and 10% of the final hybridomas consist of antibody-secreting cells (Fig. 3.1). Techniques are available to identify the correct antibody-secreting hybridoma cell, cloning or propagating that cell into large populations with subsequent large formation of the desired antibody. These cells may be frozen and later re-used.

Monoclonal antibodies have now gained wide application in many diagnostic techniques which require a high degree of specificity. Specific monoclonal antibodies have been combined into test kits for diagnostic purposes in health care, in plant and animal agriculture, and in food manufacture. Monoclonal antibodies may also be used in the future as antibody therapy to carry cytotoxic drugs to the site of cancer cells. In the fermentation industry they are already widely used as affinity ligands to bind and purify expensive products.

Since the development of the first monoclonal antibody the methodology has developed from a purely scientific tool into one of the fastest expanding fields of biotechnology, which has revolutionised, expanded and diversified the diagnostic industry. The monoclonal-antibody market is expected to continue to grow at a very high rate and, in health care alone, the anticipated annual world market could be several billion US dollars over the next decade. It is undoubtedly one of the most commercially successful and useful areas of modern biotechnology and will be expanded on in several chapters.

3.4   Genetic engineering

Genes are the fundamental basis of all life, determine the properties of all living forms of life, and are defined segments of DNA. Because the DNA structure and composition of all living forms is essentially the same, any technology that can isolate, change or reproduce a gene is likely to have an impact on almost every aspect of society.

Genetic recombination, as occurs during normal sexual reproduction, consists of the breakage and rejoining of DNA molecules of the chromosomes, and is of fundamental importance to living organisms for the reassortment of genetic material. Genetic manipulation has been performed for centuries by selective breeding of plants and animals superimposed on natural variation. The potential for genetic variation has, thus, been limited to close taxonomic relatives.

In contrast, recombinant DNA techniques, popularly termed 'gene cloning' or 'genetic engineering', offer potentially unlimited opportunities for creating new combinations of genes which, at the moment, do not exist under natural conditions.

Genetic engineering has been defined as the formation of new combinations of heritable material by the insertion of nucleic acid molecules – produced by whatever means outside the cell – into any virus, bacterial plasmid or other vector system so as to allow their incorporation into a host organism in which they do not naturally occur but in which they are capable of continued propagation. In essence, gene technology is the modification of the genetic properties of an organism by the use of recombinant DNA technology. Genes may be viewed as the biological software and are the programs which drive the growth, development and functioning of an organism. By changing the software in a precise and controlled manner, it becomes possible to produce desired changes in the characteristics of the organism.

These techniques allow the splicing of DNA molecules of quite diverse origin and, when combined with techniques of genetic transformation, etc., facilitate the introduction of foreign DNA into other organisms. The foreign DNA or gene construct is introduced into the genome of the recipient organism host in such a way that the total genome of the host is unchanged except for the manipulated gene(s).

Thus DNA can be isolated from cells of plants, animals or microorganisms (the donors) and can be fragmented into groups of one or more genes. Such fragments can then be coupled to another piece of DNA (the *vector*) and then passed into the host or recipient cell, becoming part of the genetic complement of the new host. The host cell can then be propagated in mass to form novel genetic properties and chemical abilities that were unattainable by conventional ways of selective breeding or mutation. While traditional plant and animal genetical breeding techniques also change the genetic code, it is achieved in a less direct and controlled manner. Genetic engineering will now enable the breeder to select the particular gene required for a desired characteristic and modify only that gene.

Although much work to date has involved bacteria, the techniques are evolving at an astonishing rate and ways have been developed for introducing DNA into other organisms such as yeasts and plant and animal cell cultures. Provided that the genetic material transferred in this manner can replicate and be expressed in the new cell type, there are virtually no limits to the range of organisms with new properties which could be produced by genetic engineering. Life forms containing 'foreign' DNA are termed '*transgenic*' and will be discussed in more detail in chapter 10.

These methods potentially allow totally new functions to be added to the capabilities of organisms, and open up vistas for the genetic engineering of industrial microorganisms and agricultural plants and animals which are quite breathtaking in their scope. This is undoubtedly the most significant new technology in modern bioscience and biotechnology. In industrial microbiology it will permit the production in microorganisms of a wide range of hitherto unachievable products such as human and animal proteins and enzymes such as insulin and chymosin (rennet); in medicine better vaccines, hormones and improved therapy of diseases; in agriculture improved plants and animals for productivity, quality of products, disease resistance, etc; in food production improved quality, flavour, taste and safety; and in environmental aspects a wide range of benefits such as pollution control can be expected. It should be noted that genetic engineering is a way of doing things rather than an end in itself. Genetic engineering will add to, rather than displace, traditional ways of developing products. However, there are many who view genetic engineering as a transgression of normal life processes that goes well beyond normal evolution. These concerns will be discussed in chapter 14.

Genetic engineering holds the potential to extend the range and power of almost every aspect of biotechnology. In microbial technology these techniques will be widely used to improve existing microbial processes by improving the stability of existing cultures and eliminating unwanted side-products. It is confidently anticipated that, within this decade, recombinant DNA techniques will form the basis of new strains of microorganisms with new and unusual metabolic properties. In this way fermentations based on these technical advances could become competitive with petrochemicals for producing a whole range of chemical compounds, for example ethylene glycol (used in the plastics industry). In the food industry, improved strains of bacteria and fungi are now influencing such traditional processes as baking and cheese-making and bringing greater control and reproducibility of flavour and texture.

A full understanding of the working concepts of recombinant DNA technology requires a good knowledge of molecular biology. A brief explanation will be attempted here but readers are advised to consult some of the many excellent texts that are available in this field.

The basic molecular techniques for the *in vitro* transfer and expression of foreign DNA in a host cell (*gene transfer technology*) include isolating, cutting and joining molecules of DNA, inserting into a vector (carrying) molecule that can be stably retained in the host cell.

These techniques may be defined thus:

Isolation and purification of nucleic acids. Nucleic acids from most organisms can now be routinely extracted and purified by means of a range of biochemical techniques (Fig. 3.2).

Cutting and splicing DNA. The most significant advances towards the construction of hybrid DNA molecules *in vitro* have come from the discovery that site-specific *restriction endonuclease enzymes* produce specific DNA fragments that can be joined to any similarly treated DNA molecule using another enzyme, *DNA ligase*. Restriction enzymes are present in a wide

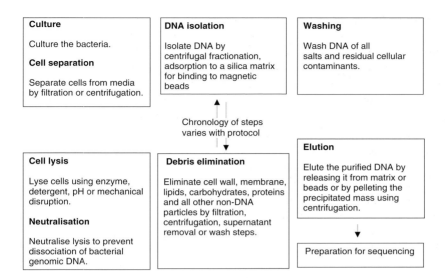

Culture	DNA isolation	Washing
Culture the bacteria. **Cell separation** Separate cells from media by filtration or centrifugation.	Isolate DNA by centrifugal fractionation, adsorption to a silica matrix for binding to magnetic beads	Wash DNA of all salts and residual cellular contaminants.

Chronology of steps
varies with protocol

Cell lysis	Debris elimination	Elution
Lyse cells using enzyme, detergent, pH or mechanical disruption. **Neutralisation** Neutralise lysis to prevent dissociation of bacterial genomic DNA.	Eliminate cell wall, membrane, lipids, carbohydrates, proteins and all other non-DNA particles by filtration, centrifugation, supernatant removal or wash steps.	Elute the purified DNA by releasing it from matrix or beads or by pelleting the precipitated mass using centrifugation.

Preparation for sequencing

Fig. 3.2 Diagram of a typical series of sample preparation steps required for DNA purification from bacterial cells (from Wells and Herron, 2002).

range of bacteria and can distinguish between DNA from their own cells and foreign DNA by recognising certain sequence of nucleotides. There are techniques available for breaking open a length of DNA into shorter fragments which contain a number of genes determined by the enzyme used. Such DNA fragments can then be separated from each other on the basis of differing molecular weights, and can subsequently be joined together in a number of ways, provided that the ends are complementary. The sources of DNA can be quite different, giving an opportunity to replicate the DNA biologically by inserting it into other cells.

The composite molecules into which DNA has been inserted have also been termed 'DNA chimeras' because of the analogy with the Chimera of mythology – a creature with the head of a lion, the body of a goat and the tail of a serpent.

The vector or carrier system. Two broad categories of vector molecules have been developed as vehicles for gene transfer, namely *plasmids* (small units of DNA distinct from chromosomes) and *bacteriophages* (or bacterial viruses). Vector molecules will normally exist within a cell in an independent or extra-chromosomal form, not becoming part of the chromosomal system of the organism. Vector molecules should be capable of entering the host cell and replicating within it. Ideally, the vector should be small, easily prepared and must contain at least one site where integration of foreign DNA will not destroy an essential function. Plasmids will undoubtedly offer the greatest potential in biotechnology and have been found in an increasingly wide range of organisms, e.g. bacteria, yeasts and mould fungi; they have been mostly studied in gram-negative bacteria.

Introduction of vector DNA recombinants. The new recombinant DNA can now be introduced into the host cell by transformations (the direct uptake of DNA by a cell from its environment) or transductions (DNA transferred from one organism to another by way of a carrier or vector system) and, if acceptable, the new DNA will be cloned with the propagation of the host cell.

Novel methods of ensuring DNA uptake into cells include *electroporation* and *mechanical particle delivery* or *biolistics*. Electroporation is a process of creating transient pores in the cell membrane by application of a pulsed electric field. Creation of such pores in a membrane allows the introduction of foreign molecules such as DNA, RNA, antibodies, drugs, etc., into the cell cytoplasm. Development of this technology has arisen from synergy of biophysics, bioengineering and cell and molecular biology. While the technique is now widely used to create transgenic microorganisms, plants and animals, it is also being increasingly used for the application of therapeutics and gene therapy. The mechanical particle delivery or 'gene gun' methods deliver DNA on microscopic particles into target tissue or cells. This process is increasingly used to introduce new genes into a range of bacterial, fungal, plant and mammalian species and has become a main method of choice for genetic engineering of many plant species including rice, corn, wheat, cotton and soybean.

The strategies involved in genetic engineering are summarised in Table 3.1 and Fig. 3.3.

Although the theory underlying the exchange of genetic information between unrelated organisms and their propagation is becoming better understood, difficulties still persist at the level of some applications. Further research is required before such exchanges become commonplace and the host organisms are propagated in large quantities.

Early studies on genetic engineering were mainly carried out with the bacterium *Escherichia coli* but, increasingly, other bacteria, yeast and filamentous fungi have been used. Mammalian systems have been increasingly developed using the simian virus (SV40) and oncogenes (genes that cause cancer), while several successful methods are available for plant cells, in particular the

Table 3.1. Strategies involved in genetic engineering

Strategy	Method
Formation of DNA fragments	Extracted DNA can be cut into small sequences by specific enzymes – restriction endonucleases found in many species of bacteria.
Splicing of DNA into vectors	The small sequences of DNA can be joined or spliced into the vector DNA molecules by an enzyme DNA ligase, creating an artificial DNA molecule.
Introduction of vectors into host cells	The vectors are either viruses or plasmids, and are replicons and can exist in an extra-chromosomal state; they can be transferred normally by transduction or transformation.
Selection of newly acquired DNA	Selection and ultimate characterisation of the recombinant clone.

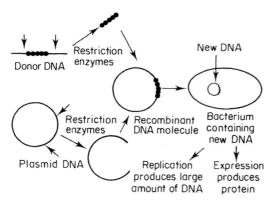

Fig. 3.3 Recombinant DNA: the technique of recombining genes from one species with those of another.

Agrobacterium system (Chapter 10). Thus, in the last four decades, molecular biology has formulated evidence for the unity of genetic systems together with the basic mechanisms that regulate cell function. Genetic engineering has confirmed the unity of the living world, demonstrating that all living creatures are built of molecules that are more or less identical. Thus, the diversity of life forms on this planet derives from small changes in the regulatory systems that control the expression of genes.

3.5   The polymerase chain reaction and DNA sequencing

Two molecular biology techniques in recent years have revolutionised the availability of DNA data, namely the polymerase chain reaction (PCR) and the development of automated DNA sequencing. A PCR is basically a technique which allows the selective amplification of any fragment of DNA provided that the DNA sequences flanking the fragment are known – described as a technique which finds a needle in a haystack and then produces a haystack of needles by specific amplification! The inventor of PCR, Kary Mullis, shared the Nobel Prize in Chemistry in 1993.

The PCR process relies on the sequence of 'base pairs' along the length of the two strands that make the complete DNA molecule. In DNA there are four deoxynucleotides derived from the four bases, adenine (A), thymine (T), guanine (G) and cytosine (C). The strands or polymers that comprise the DNA molecule are held to each other by hydrogen bonds between the base pairs. In this arrangement, A only binds to T while G only binds to C, and this unique system folds the entire molecule into the now well-recognised double-helix structure.

PCR involves three processing steps: *denaturation, annealing* and then *extension* by DNA polymerase (Fig. 3.4a, b). In Step 1, the double-stranded DNA is heated (95–98°C) and separates into two complementary single strands. In Step 2 (60°C), the synthetic oligonucleotide primers (chemically synthesised short-chain nucleotides) – short sequences of nucleotides (usually about 20 nucleotide base pairs long) – are added and bind to the single strands in places where the strand's DNA complements their own. In Step 3 (37°C), the primers are extended by DNA polymerase in the presence of all four deoxynucleoside triphosphates, resulting in the synthesis of new DNA strands that are complementary to the template strands. The completion of the three steps comprises a cycle and the real power of PCR is that, with 25–30 cycles, this experimental synthesis leads to massive amplification of DNA which can then be used for analytical purposes. A major recent advance has been the development of automated thermal cyclers (PCR machines), which allow the entire PCR to be performed automatically in several hours.

PCR was first patented in 1987 and then commercialised by the American Cetus Corporation in 1988. However, in 1991, Hoffman La Roche and Perkin Elmer purchased the full operating rights of PCR for $300 million. The applications of PCR increase almost daily and include: molecular biology/genetic engineering, infectious and parasitic disease diagnosis, human genetic disease diagnosis, forensic validation, plant and animal breeding, and environmental

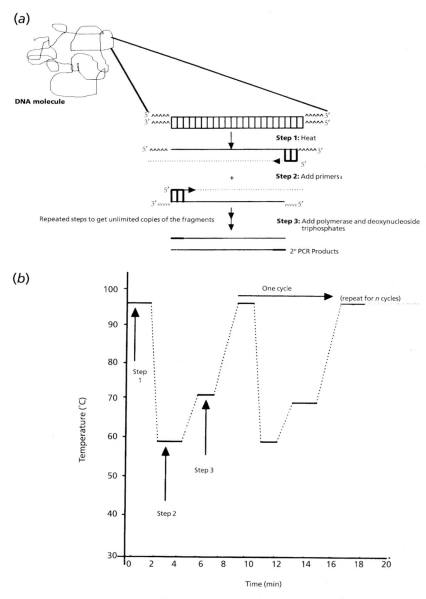

(a)

DNA molecule

Step 1: Heat

Step 2: Add primers ↓

+

Repeated steps to get unlimited copies of the fragments

Step 3: Add polymerase and deoxynucleoside triphosphates

2^n PCR Products

(b)

One cycle

(repeat for n cycles)

Step 1

Step 3

Step 2

Temperature (°C)

Time (min)

Fig. 3.4 (a) The polymerase chain reaction. The double-stranded DNA is heated and separates into two single strands. The synthetic oligonucleotide primers then bind to their complementary sequence and are extended in the direction of the arrows, giving a new strand of DNA identical to the template's original partner; (b) PCR temperature cycling profile (see Graham, 1994).

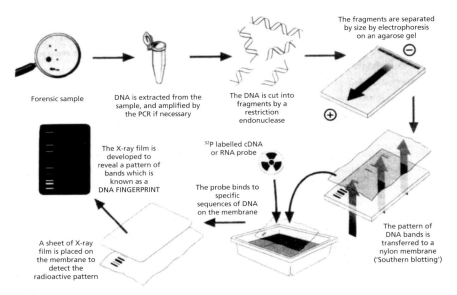

Forensic sample

DNA is extracted from the sample, and amplified by the PCR if necessary

The DNA is cut into fragments by a restriction endonuclease

The fragments are separated by size by electrophoresis on an agarose gel

The pattern of DNA bands is transferred to a nylon membrane ('Southern blotting')

The probe binds to specific sequences of DNA on the membrane

^{32}P labelled cDNA or RNA probe

The X-ray film is developed to reveal a pattern of bands which is known as a DNA FINGERPRINT

A sheet of X-ray film is placed on the membrane to detect the radioactive pattern

Fig. 3.5   DNA fingerprinting (from Grainger and Madden, 1993).

monitoring. PCR has been extensively used in the well-known procedure of genetic or DNA fingerprinting, the fallibility of which is now being challenged in courts of law (Fig. 3.5).

While PCR is finding considerable and unique use in archaeology, it is doubtful whether we will ever be able to resurrect woolly mammoths and dinosaurs from ancient animal remains, as recently epitomised in Michael Crighton's *Jurassic Park*.

Genomes of all organisms consist of millions of repetitions of the four nucleotides – C, G, A and T. In humans, there are over 3000 million nucleotides. Analysing the sequence of the nucleotides (*DNA sequencing*) has become a critically useful technique for the identification, analysis and directed manipulation of genomic DNA. Originally, methods of separation and identification relied upon gel electrophoresis and autoradiography. However, recent developments in sequencing technology have allowed the process to be automated and greatly speeded up. Fluorescent dye-labelled substrates are used, which allow the use of a laser-induced fluorescent detection system. In many applications automated sequencers can produce over 1000 base pairs of sequences from overnight operations. There are now publicly available databases such as GenBank, which provide numerous online services for identifying, aligning and comparing sequences. Individual chromosomes contain many thousands of sequences, some of which are organised into genes while others appear to be merely flanking or spacer regions.

3.6   Genomics and proteomics

The genetic heritable material of living cells resides with the nucleic acids of the chromosomes and is termed the '*genome*'. Arising from the previously described techniques, it was possible in 1995 to determine the first complete genome or DNA sequence of a free-living organism, the bacterium *Haemophilus influenzae*. Since then, a considerable number of prokaryotes, the yeast *Saccharomyces cerevisiae*, the fruit-fly *Drosophila melanogaster* and the plant *Arabidopsis thaliana* have been sequenced. However, the major event in molecular genetics was the elucidation of the human genome sequence in 2001. The academic and commercial drive to decipher the human genome was largely driven by a belief that major medical developments would unfold. Consequently, many billions of dollars have been spent to achieve this momentous level of genomic knowledge. While there has been much hype concerning the ethical and commercial implications of these discoveries, this is only the beginning of the understanding of the real functional activity within cells, in tissues and in whole organisms. Throughout this last decade of genomic research there has been insufficient emphasis on other aspects of cellular organisation and much ill-judged scientific belief that the enigma of cell function in health and disease could be understood solely through knowledge of genes alone.

Biochemical studies over many decades have shown that cellular activity is achieved through a vast array of signalling and regulatory and metabolic pathways, each involving many specific molecules. There still exists a vast gulf between our understanding of individual molecular mechanisms and pathways and how they are integrated into an orderly *homeostatic* system.

Major molecular biology attention has now moved dramatically to the study of the *proteome* – the collective body of proteins made within an organism's cells and tissues. While the genome supplies the recipes for making the cell's proteins, it is the proteome that represents the bricks and mortar of the cells and carries out the cellular functions. The proteome is infinitely more complicated than the genome. While a cell will have only one genome, it can have many proteomes. The DNA alphabet is composed of four chained bases, while proteins, in contrast, are constructed from approximately 20 amino acids. While the genes through transcription determine the sequence of amino acids in a protein, it is not totally clear what the protein does and how it interacts with other proteins. Unlike genes which are linear, proteins fold into three-dimensional structures which are difficult to predict. The proteome is extremely dynamic, and minor alterations in the external or internal environment can modify proteome function. Understanding proteomics should give a better holistic view of cellular metabolism.

The dominant biochemical approach to proteomics combines two-dimensional polyacrylamide gel electrophoresis (2D-PAGE), which separates, maps and quanitifies proteins, with mass spectrometry (MS)-based sequencing techniques which identify both the amino acid sequences of proteins and the post-translationary molecular additions. Proteomics will relate to genomic databases to assist protein identification and consequently will indicate which genes within the database are important in specific conditions. The two areas of genomics and proteomics must have a strong synergistic relationship. The potential of proteomics to identify and compare complex protein profiles is now generating highly accurate but sensitive molecular fingerprints of proteins present in human body fluids at a given time. These may well offer early markers of diseased status in the human system. Such molecular medicine could well be one of the most remarkable achievements of biotechnology of this century.

The ability to clone DNA or manipulate genes and to obtain successful expression in an organism is nowadays a core technology of quite unparalleled importance in modern bioscience and biotechnology. The expression and acceptance of genetic engineering in the context of biotechnology, where novel gene pools can be created and expressed in large quantities, will offer outstanding opportunities for the well-being of humanity.

3.7   Potential laboratory biohazards of genetic engineering

The early studies on gene manipulation provoked wide discussion and considerable concern at the possible risks that could arise with certain types of experiment. Thus it was believed by some that the construction of recombinant DNA molecules and their insertion into microorganisms could create novel organisms which might inadvertently be released from the laboratory and become a biohazard to humans or the environment. In contrast, others considered that newly synthesised organisms with their additional genetic material would not be able to compete with the normal strains present in nature. The present views of gene manipulation studies are becoming more moderate as experiments have shown that this work can proceed within a strict safety code when required, involving physical and biological containment of the organism.

The standards of containment enforced in the early years of recombinant DNA studies were unnecessarily restrictive and there has been a steady relaxation of the regulations governing much of the routine genetic engineering activities. However, for many types of study – particularly with pathogenic microorganisms – the standards will remain stringent. Thus, for strict physical containment, laboratories involved in this type of study must have highly skilled personnel and correct physical containment equipment, e.g. negative pressure laboratories, autoclaves and safety cabinets.

Biological containment can be achieved or enhanced by selecting non-pathogenic organisms as the cloning agents of foreign DNA or by the deliberate genetic manipulation of a microorganism to reduce the probability of survival and propagation in the environment. *Escherichia coli*, a bacterium which is extremely prevalent in the intestinal tracts of warm-blooded and cold-blooded animals as well as in humans, is the most widely used cloning agent. To offset the risk of this cloning agent becoming a danger in the environment, a special strain of *E. coli* has been constructed by genetic manipulation which incorporates many fail-safe features. This strain can only grow under special laboratory conditions and there is no possibility that it can constitute a biohazard if it escapes out of the laboratory.

The government-controlled Health and Safety Executive controls and monitors recombinant DNA work within the UK. This committee seeks advice from the Genetic Manipulation Advisory Group (GMAG), who formulate realistic procedural guidelines which, in general, have proved widely acceptable to the experimenting scientific community. Most other advanced scientific nations involved in recombinant DNA studies have set up similar advisory committees. The deliberate releasing of genetically manipulated organisms to the environment is discussed in Chapter 14.

4

Bioprocess/fermentation technology

4.1 Introduction

Bioprocess or fermentation technology is an important component of most 'old' and 'new' biotechnology processes and will normally involve complete living cells (microbe, mammalian or plant), organelles or enzymes as the biocatalyst and will aim to bring about specific chemical and/or physical changes in organic materials (the medium). In order to be viable in any specific industrial context, bioprocessing must possess advantages over competing methods of production such as chemical technology. In practice, many bioprocessing techniques will be used industrially because they are the only practical way in which a specific product can be made (e.g. vaccines, antibiotics).

The very beginnings of fermentation technology, or as it is now better recognised, 'bioprocess technology', were derived in part from the use of microorganisms for the production of foods such as cheeses, yoghurts, sauerkraut, fermented pickles and sausages, soy sauce, and other Oriental products, and beverages such as beers, wines and derived spirits (Table 4.1). In many cases, the present-day production processes for such products are still remarkably similar. These forms of bioprocessing were long viewed as arts or crafts but are now increasingly subjected to the full array of modern science and technology. Paralleling these useful product formations was the identification of the roles that microorganisms could play in removing obnoxious and unhealthful wastes, which has resulted in worldwide service industries involved in water purification, effluent treatment and solid waste management (Chapter 9).

Bioprocessing in its many forms involves a multitude of complex enzyme-catalysed reactions within specific cellular systems, and these reactions are

Table 4.1. Fermentation products according to industrial sectors

Sector	Products/activities
Chemicals	
Organic (bulk)	Ethanol, acetone, butanol
	Organic acids (citric, itaconic)
Organic (fine)	Enzymes
	Perfumeries
	Polymers (mainly polysaccharides)
Inorganic	Metal beneficiation, bioaccumulation and leaching (Cu, U)
Pharmaceuticals	Antibiotics
	Diagnostic agents (enzymes, monoclonal antibodies)
	Enzyme inhibitors
	Steroids
	Vaccines
Energy	Ethanol (gasohol)
	Methane (biogas)
	Biomass
Food	Dairy products (cheeses, yoghurts, fish and meat products)
	Beverages (alcoholic, tea and coffee)
	Baker's yeast
	Food additives (antioxidants, colours, flavours, stabilisers)
	Novel foods (soy sauce, tempeh, miso)
	Mushroom products
	Amino acids, vitamins
	Starch products
	Glucose and high-fructose syrups
	Functional modifications of proteins, pectins
Agriculture	Animal feedstuffs (SCP)
	Veterinary vaccines
	Ensilage and composting processes
	Microbial pesticides
	Rhizobium and other N-fixing bacterial inoculants
	Mycorrhizal inoculants
	Plant cell and tissue culture (vegetative propagation, embryo production, genetic improvement)

Adapted from Bull *et al.* (1982).

critically dependent on the physical and chemical conditions that exist in their immediate environment. Successful bioprocessing will only occur when all the essential factors are brought together.

Although the traditional forms of bioprocess technology related to foods and beverages still represent the major commercial bioproducts, new products are increasingly being derived from microbial and mammalian fermentations, namely:

(1) in the overproduction of essential primary metabolites, e.g. acetic and lactic acids, glycerol, acetone, butyl alcohol, organic acids, amino acids, vitamins and polysaccharides;

(2) in the production of secondary metabolites (metabolites that do not appear to have an obvious role in the metabolism of the producer organism), e.g. penicillin, streptomycin, cephalosporin, gibberellins;

(3) in the production of many forms of industrially useful enzymes, e.g. exocellular enzymes such as amylases, pectinases and proteases and intracellular enzymes such as invertase, asparaginase and restriction endonucleases;

(4) in the production of monoclonal antibodies, vaccines and novel recombinant products, e.g. therapeutic proteins.

All of these products now command large industrial markets and are essential to modern society (Table 4.1).

More recently, bioprocess technology is increasingly using cells derived from higher plants and animals to produce many important products. Plant cell culture is largely aimed at secondary product formations such as flavours, perfumes and drugs, while mammalian cell culture has been concerned with vaccine and antibody formation and the recombinant production of protein molecules such as interferon, interleukins and erythropoietin.

The future market growth of these bioproducts is largely assured because, with limited exceptions, most cannot be produced economically by other chemical processes. It will also be possible to make further economies in production by genetically engineering organisms to higher or unique productivities and utilising new technological advances in processing. The advantages of producing organic products by biological, as opposed to purely chemical, methods are listed in Table 4.2.

The product formation stages in bioprocess technology are essentially very similar regardless of the organism selected, the medium used and the product formed. In all examples, large numbers of cells are grown under defined controlled conditions. The organisms must be cultivated *and* motivated to form the desired products by means of a physical/technical containment system (*bioreactor*) and the correct medium composition and environmental

Table 4.2. Advantages and disadvantages of producing organic compounds by biological rather than chemical means

Advantages	Disadvantages
Complex molecules such as proteins and antibodies cannot be produced by chemical means.	The product can be easily contaminated with foreign unwanted microorganisms, etc.
Bioconversions give higher yields.	The desired product will usually be present in a complex product mixture requiring separation.
Biological systems operate at lower temperatures, near neutral pH, etc.	There is a need to provide, handle and dispose of large volumes of water.
There is much greater specificity of catalytic reaction.	Bioprocesses are usually extremely slow when compared with conventional chemical processes.
Exclusive production of an isomeric compound can be achieved.	

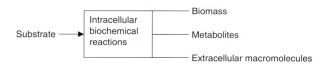

Fig. 4.1 The biotechnology process.

growth-regulating parameters such as temperature and aeration. Optimisation of the bioprocess spans both the bio- and the technical systems. The proper exploitation of an organism's potential to form distinct products of defined quality *and* in large amounts requires a detailed knowledge of the biochemical mechanisms of product formation.

Bioprocessing in its many forms is catalysed with each respective cellular system by a large number of intracellular biochemical reactions. Substrates derived from the medium are converted into primary and secondary products, intra- and extracellular macromolecules, and biomass components such as DNA, RNA, proteins and carbohydrates (Fig. 4.1).

These reactions will be dependent on the physical and chemical parameters that exist in their immediate environments.

The same apparatus with modifications can be used to produce an enzyme, an antibiotic, an amino acid or a single cell protein. In its simplest form, the

Table 4.3. Examples of products in different categories in biotechnological industries

Category	Example
Cell mass[a]	Baker's yeast, SCP
Cell components[b]	Intracellular proteins
Biosynthetic products[b]	Antibiotics, vitamins, amino and organic acids
Catabolic products[a]	Ethanol, methane, lactic acid
Bioconversion[a]	High-fructose corn syrup, 6-aminopenicillanic acid
Waste treatment	Activated sludge, anaerobic digestion

[a] Typically, conversion of feedstock cost-intensive processes.
[b] Typically, recovery cost-intensive process.

bioprocess can be viewed merely by mixing the microorganisms with a nutrient broth and allowing the components to react, e.g. mixing yeast cells with a sugar solution to give alcohol. More advanced and sophisticated processes operating on a large scale need to control the entire system so that the bioprocess can proceed efficiently and be readily and exactly repeated with the same amounts of raw materials and inoculum (the particular organism) to produce precisely the same amount of product.

All biotechnological processes are essentially performed within containment systems or bioreactors. Large numbers of cells are invariably involved in these processes and the bioreactor ensures their close involvement with the correct medium and conditions for growth and product formation. It also should restrict the release of the cells into the environment. A main function of a bioreactor is to minimise the cost of producing a product or service. Examples of the diverse product categories produced industrially in bioreactors are given in Table 4.3.

4.2 Principles of microbial growth

The growth of organisms may be seen as the increase of cell material expressed in terms of mass or cell number and results from a highly complicated and coordinated series of enzymatically catalysed biological steps. Growth will be dependent both on the availability and transport of necessary nutrients to the cell and subsequent uptake and on environmental parameters such as temperature, pH and aeration being optimally maintained.

The quantity of biomass or specific cellular component in a bioreactor can be determined gravimetrically (by dry weight, wet weight, DNA or protein)

Table 4.4. Approximate size of cells used in biotechnology processes

Cell type	Size (μm)
Bacterial cells	1 × 2
Yeast cells	7 × 10
Mammalian cells	40 × 40
Plant cells	100 × 100

or numerically for unicellular systems (by number of cells). Doubling time refers to the period of time required for the doubling in the weight of biomass, while generation time relates to the period necessary for the doubling of cell numbers. Average doubling times increase with increasing cell size (Table 4.4) and complexity, e.g. doubling time for bacteria is 0.25–1 h; yeast 1–2 h; mould fungi 2–6.5 h; plant cells 20–70 h; and mammalian cells 20–48 h.

In normal practice an organism will seldom have totally ideal conditions for unlimited growth; rather, growth will be dependent on a limiting factor, for example an essential nutrient. As the concentration of this factor drops, so also will the growth potential of the organism decrease.

In biotechnological processes there are three main ways of growing microorganisms in the bioreactor: batch, semi-continuous or continuous. Within the bioreactor, reactions can occur with static or agitated cultures, in the presence or absence of oxygen, and in liquid or low-moisture conditions (e.g. on solid substrates). The microorganisms can be free or can be attached to surfaces by immobilisation or by natural adherence.

In a *batch culture*, the microorganisms are inoculated into a fixed volume of medium and, as growth takes place, nutrients are consumed and products of growth (biomass, metabolites) accumulate. The nutrient environment within the bioreactor is continuously changing and, thus, in turn, enforcing changes to cell metabolism. Eventually, cell multiplication ceases because of exhaustion or limitation of nutrient(s) and accumulation of toxic excreted waste products.

The complex nature of batch growth of microorganisms is shown in Fig. 4.2. The initial *lag phase* is a time of no apparent growth but actual biochemical analyses show metabolic turnover, indicating that the cells are in the process of adapting to the environmental conditions and that new growth will eventually begin. There is then a *transient acceleration* phase as the inoculum begins to grow, which is quickly followed by the *exponential phase*. In the exponential phase microbial growth proceeds at the maximum possible rate for that organism with nutrients in excess, ideal environmental parameters

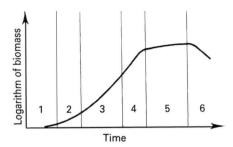

Fig. 4.2   Growth characteristics in a batch culture of a microorganism. 1, lag phase; 2, transient acceleration; 3, exponential phase; 4, deceleration phase; 5, stationary phase; 6, death phase.

and growth inhibitors absent. However, in batch cultivations exponential growth is of limited duration and, as nutrient conditions change, growth rate decreases, entering the *deceleration phase*, to be followed by the *stationary phase*, when overall growth can no longer be obtained owing to nutrient exhaustion. The final phase of the cycle is the *death phase*, when growth rate has ceased. Most biotechnological batch processes are stopped before this stage because of decreasing metabolism and cell lysis.

In industrial usage, batch cultivation has been carried out to optimise organism or biomass production and then to allow the organism to perform specific biochemical transformations such as end-product formation (e.g. amino acids, enzymes) or decomposition of substances (sewage treatment, bioremediation). Many important products such as antibiotics are optimally formed during the stationary phase of the growth cycle in batch cultivation.

However, there are means of prolonging the life of a batch culture and thus increasing the yield by various substrate feed methods:

(1) by the gradual addition of concentrated components of the nutrient, e.g. carbohydrates, so increasing the volume of the culture (*fed batch*) – used for the industrial production of baker's yeast;
(2) by the addition of medium to the culture (*perfusion*) and withdrawal of an equal volume of used cell-free medium – used in mammalian cell cultivations.

In contrast to batch conditions, the practice of *continuous cultivation* gives near balanced growth with little fluctuation of nutrients, metabolites or cell numbers or biomass. This practice depends on fresh medium entering a batch system at the exponential phase of growth with a corresponding withdrawal

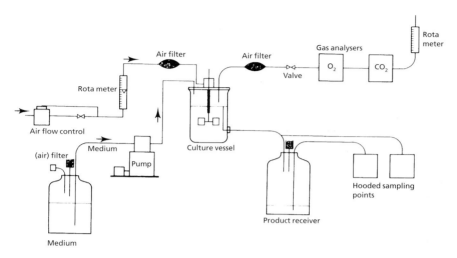

Fig. 4.3 A simple laboratory fermenter operating on a continuous-cultivation basis.

of medium *plus* cells. Continuous methods of cultivation will permit organisms to grow under steady state (unchanging) conditions in which growth occurs at a constant rate and in a constant environment. In a completely mixed continuous-culture system, sterile medium is passed into the bioreactor (Fig. 4.3) at a steady flow rate and culture broth (medium, waste products and organisms) emerges from it at the same rate, keeping the volume of the total culture in the bioreactor constant. Factors such as pH and the concentrations of nutrients and metabolic products, which inevitably change during batch cultivation, can be held near constant in continuous cultivations. In industrial practice continuously operated systems are of limited use and include only single cell protein (SCP) and ethanol productions and some forms of waste water treatment processes. However, for many reasons (Table 4.5) batch cultivation systems represent the dominant form of industrial usage. The full range of cultivation methods for microorganisms is shown in Table 4.6.

Microorganisms utilised in industrial biotechnology processes are normally held in great secrecy by the commercial companies. They have been derived from extensive selection processes and optimised by culture development for optimum productivity. Methods have been developed for long-term storage to maintain culture stability and productivity. National and International Culture Collection Centres conserve a wide range of microbial cultures, which provide an organism base for biosystematics and support bioscience and biotechnology research and development.

Table 4.5. Advantages of batch and fed-batch culture techniques in industry

(1) The products may be required only in relatively small quantities at any given time.
(2) Market needs may be intermittent.
(3) The shelf-life of certain products is short.
(4) High product concentration is required in broth to optimise downstream processing operations.
(5) Some metabolic products are produced only during the stationary phase of the growth cycle.
(6) The instability of some production strains requires their regular renewal.
(7) Continuous processes can offer many technical difficulties.

4.3   The bioreactor

Bioreactors are the containment vehicles of any biotechnology-based production process, be it for brewing, organic or amino acids, antibiotics, enzymes or vaccines or for bioremediation. For each biotechnology process the most suitable containment system must be designed to give the correct environment for optimising the growth and metabolic activity of the biocatalyst. Bioreactors range from simple stirred or non-stirred open containers to complex aseptic integrated systems involving varying levels of advanced computer control (Fig. 4.4).

Bioreactors occur in two distinct types (Fig. 4.4). In the first instance they are primarily non-aseptic systems where it is not absolutely essential to operate with entirely pure cultures, e.g. brewing, effluent disposal systems, while in the second type aseptic conditions are a prerequisite for successful product formation, e.g. antibiotics, vitamins, polysaccharides. This type of process involves considerable challenges on the part of engineering construction and operation.

The physical form of many of the most widely used bioreactors has not altered much over the past 40 years; however, in recent years, novel forms of bioreactors have been developed to suit the needs of specific bioprocesses, and such innovations are finding increasingly specialised roles in bioprocess technology (Fig. 4.4).

In all forms of fermentation the ultimate aim is to ensure that all parts of the system are subject to the same conditions. Within the bioreactor the microorganisms are suspended in the aqueous nutrient medium containing the necessary substrates for growth of the organism and required product

Table 4.6. Characteristics of cultivation methods

Type of culture	Operational characteristics	Application
Solid	Simple, cheap selection of colonies from single cell possible; process control limited	Maintenance of strains, genetic studies; production of enzymes; composting
Film	Various types of bioreactors; trickling filter, rotating disc, packed bed, sponge reactor, rotating tube	Waste-water treatment, monolayer culture (animal cells); bacterial leaching; vinegar production
Submerged homogeneous distribution of cells; batch	'Spontaneous' reaction, various types of reactor: stirred tank bioreactor, air lift, loop, deep shaft, etc; agitation by stirrers, air, liquid process control for physical parameters possible; less for chemical and biological parameters	Standard type of cultivation: antibiotics, solvents, acids, etc.
Fed-batch	Simple method for control of regulatory effects, e.g. glucose repression	Production of baker's yeast
Continuous one-stage homogeneous	Proper control of reaction; excellent role for kinetic and regulatory studies; higher costs for experiment; problem of aseptic operation, the need for highly trained operators	Few cases of application in industrial scale; production of SCP; waste water treatment

formation. All nutrients, including oxygen, must be provided to diffuse into each cell and waste products such as heat, CO_2 and waste metabolites removed.

The concentration of the nutrients in the vicinity of the organism must be held within a definite range since low values will limit the rate of organism metabolism while excessive concentrations can be toxic. Biological reactions run most efficiently within optimum ranges of environmental parameters, and in biotechnological processes these conditions must be provided on a micro-scale so that each cell is equally provided for. When the large scale of many bioreactor systems is considered, it will be realised how difficult it is to achieve

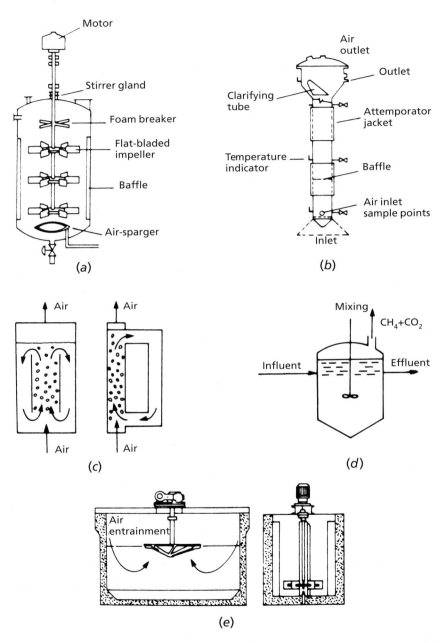

Fig. 4.4   Various forms of bioreactor. (a) Stirred tank bioreactor; (b) tower reactor; (c) loop (recycle) bioreactor; (d) anaerobic digester or bioreactor; (e) activated sludge bioreactor. (a) and (b) reproduced by permission from Kristiansen and Chamberlain (1983).

Table 4.7. Standards of materials used in sophisticated fermenter design

---

(1) All materials coming into contact with the solutions entering the bioreactor or the actual organism culture must be corrosion resistant to prevent trace-metal contamination of the process.
(2) The materials must be non-toxic so that slight dissolution of the material or components does not inhibit culture growth.
(3) The materials of the bioreactor must withstand repeated sterilisation with high-pressure steam.
(4) The bioreactor stirrer system, entry ports and end plates must be easily machinable and sufficiently rigid so as not to be deformed or broken under mechanical stress.
(5) Visual inspection of the medium and culture is advantageous; transparent materials should be used wherever possible.

---

these conditions in a whole population. It is here that the skills of the process or biochemical engineer and the microbiologist must come together.

Fermentation reactions are multiphase, involving a gas phase (containing N_2, O_2 and CO_2), one or more liquid phases (aqueous medium and liquid substrate) and a solid microphase (the microorganisms and, possibly, solid substrates). All phases must be kept in close contact to achieve rapid mass and heat transfer. In a perfectly mixed bioreactor, all reactants entering the system must be immediately mixed and uniformly distributed to ensure homogeneity inside the reactor.

To achieve optimisation of the bioreactor system, the following operating guidelines must be closely adhered to:

(1) The bioreactor should be designed to exclude entrance of contaminating organisms as well as containing the desired organisms;
(2) The culture volume should remain constant, i.e. no leakage or evaporation;
(3) The dissolved oxygen level must be maintained above critical levels of aeration and culture agitation for aerobic organisms;
(4) Environmental parameters such as temperature, pH, etc., must be controlled, and the culture volume must be well mixed.

The standards of materials used in the construction of sophisticated fermenters is important (Table 4.7).

Fermentation technologists seek to achieve a maximisation of culture potential by accurate control of the bioreactor environment. But still there is a great lack of true understanding of just what environmental conditions will produce an optimal yield of organism or product.

Successful bioprocessing will only occur when all the specific growth-related parameters are brought together and the information used to improve and optimise the process. For successful commercial operation of these bioprocesses, quantitative description of the cellular processes is an essential prerequisite. The two most relevant aspects, *yield* and *productivity,* are quantitative measures that will indicate how the cells convert the substrate into the product. The yield represents the amount of product obtained from the substrate while the productivity specifies the rate of product formation.

To understand and control a fermentation process it is necessary to know the state of the process over a small time increment and, further, to know how the organism responds to a set of measurable environmental conditions. Process optimisation requires accurate and rapid feedback control. In the future, the computer will be an integral part of most bioreactor systems. However, there is a lack of good sensor probes that will allow on-line analysis to be made on the chemical components of the fermentation process.

A large worldwide market exists for the development of new rapid methods for monitoring the many reactions within a bioreactor. In particular, the greatest need is for innovatory micro-electronic designs.

When endeavouring to improve existing process operations or designing, it is often advisable to set up mathematical models of the overall system. A model is a set of relationships between the variables in the system being studied. Such relationships are usually expressed in the form of mathematical equations but can also be specific as cause/effect relationships which can be used in the operation of the specific processes. The actual variables involved can be extensive but will include any parameter that is of importance for the process, and can include pH, temperature, substrate concentration, agitation, feed rate, etc.

Bioreactor configurations have changed considerably over the last few decades. The original fermentation system was a shallow tank that was agitated or stirred by manpower. From this has developed the basic aeration tower system which now dominates industrial usage. As fermentation systems were further developed, two design solutions to the problems of aeration and agitation have been implemented. The first approach uses mechanical aeration and agitation devices, with relatively high power requirements; the standard example is the stirred tank bioreactor, which is widely used throughout conventional laboratory and industrial fermentations. Such bioreactors ensure good gas/liquid mass transfer, have reasonable heat transfer, and ensure good mixing of the bioreactor contents.

The second main approach to aerobic bioreactor design uses air distribution (with low power consumption) to create forced and controlled liquid flow in a recycle or loop bioreactor. In this way the contents are subjected to a controlled recycle flow, either within the bioreactor or involving an external recycle loop. Thus stirring has been replaced by pumping, which may be mechanical or pneumatic, as in the case of the airlift bioreactor.

The CSTR consists of a cylindrical vessel with a motor-driven central shaft that supports one or several agitators, with the shaft entering either through the top or the bottom of the vessels. The aspect ratio (i.e. height-to-diameter ratio) of the vessel is 3:5 for microbial systems, while for mammalian cell culture the aspect ratios do not normally exceed 2. Sterile air is sparged into the bioreactor liquid below the bottom impeller by way of a perforated ring sparger. The speed of the impellors will be related to the degree of fragility of the cells. Mammalian cells are extremely fragile when compared with most microorganisms. In a great many of the high-value processes, the bioreactors will be operated in a batch manner under aseptic monoculture. The bioreactors can range from about 20 litres to in excess of 250 m^3 for particular processes. The initial culture expansion of the microorganisms will commence in the smallest bioreactor, and when growth is optimised, will then be transferred to a larger bioreactor, and so forth, until the final-operation bioreactor. Throughout such operations it is imperative to maintain aseptic conditions to ensure the success of the process. Bioreactors are normally sterilised prior to inoculation, and contamination must be avoided during all subsequent operations. If contamination occurs during the cultivation this will invariably lead to process failure since, more often, the contaminant can outgrow the participating monoculture.

Large amounts of organic waste waters from domestic and industrial sources are routinely treated in aerobic and anaerobic systems. Activated sludge processes are widely used for the oxidative treatment of sewage and other liquid wastes (Fig. 4.4d). Such processes use batch or continuously agitated bioreactor systems to increase the entrainment of air to optimise oxidative breakdown of the organic material. These bioreactors are large and, for optimum functioning, will have several or many agitator units to facilitate mixing and oxygen uptake. They are widely used in most municipal sewage treatment plants.

Anaerobic bioreactors or digestors have long been used to treat sewage matter. In the absence of free oxygen, certain microbial consortia are able to convert biodegradable organic material to methane, carbon dioxide and new microbial biomass. Most common anaerobic digesters work on a continuous or semi-continuous manner.

An outstanding example of methane generation is the Chinese biogas programme, where millions of family-size anaerobic bioreactors are in operation. Such bioreactors are used for the treatment of manure, human excreta, etc., producing biogas for cooking and lighting and the sanitisation of the waste, which then becomes an excellent fertiliser.

In almost all fermentation processes performed in a bioreactor there is generally a need to measure specific growth-related and environmental parameters, record them and then use the information to improve and optimise the process. Bioreactor control measurements are made in either an on-line or an off-line manner. With an on-line measurement, the sensor is placed directly with the process stream, whereas for off-line measurement a sample is removed aseptically from the process stream and analysed. Bioreactor processing is still severely limited by a shortage of reliable instruments capable of on-line measurement of important variables such as DNA, RNA, enzymes and biomass. Off-line analysis is still essential for these compounds, and since the results of these analyses are usually not available until several hours after sampling, they cannot be used for immediate control purposes. However, on-line measurement is readily available for temperature, pH, dissolved oxygen and CO_2 analyses.

The continued discovery of new products such as therapeutic drugs from microorganisms and mammalian cells will continue to depend on the development of innovative exploratory culture systems which encourage the biosynthesis of novel compounds. New miniaturised, computer-controlled incubator systems with automated analysis units are now available as single units which can perform hundreds of experiments simultaneously, thus producing a wealth of data in a short time to facilitate optimum fermentation conditions for product formation.

A new and quite novel approach involving combinatorial biology generates new products from genetically engineered microorganisms. DNA fragments or genes derived from unusual microorganisms that are not easily cultivated (recalcitrant microorganisms) can be transferred into easily cultivated or surrogate microorganisms, and the resulting mixing and matching of genes encoding biosynthetic machinery is now offering the opportunity to discover new or modified molecules or drugs. This could be of great significance in antibiotic discovery.

While most high-value biotechnological compounds such as antibiotics and therapeutic proteins are produced in monoculture under strict conditions of asepsis, there are now new avenues of research exploring product formation from mixed-culture systems. Such systems may well produce different patterns of metabolites or, indeed, novel metabolites as a result of interactions which can occur between competing microorganisms. Because of the complexity of these mixed organism processes, they have all but been ignored by the scientific community. Monoculture under aseptic conditions is totally unnatural and rarely, if ever, occurs in nature. The norm is for microorganisms to exist together in the environment and to compete and respond to substrate availability and prevailing environmental conditions.

4.4   Scale-up

Most biotechnological processes will have been identified at laboratory scale and ultimate commercial success will be dependent on the ability to scale-up the process first from laboratory to pilot plant level and then to full commercial scale. The achievement of successful process scale-up must fit within a range of physical and economic restraints. The identification of some of the controlling parameters can usually be made with laboratory-scale bioreactors (5–10 litres) and then moved to pilot-scale level. A pilot plant is, in reality, a large-scale laboratory which has been designed to give flexibility for equipment accommodation and adaptability for process operation. Pilot-plant bioreactors range from 100 liters to 10 000 litres total volume, and the larger pilot bioreactors can, on occasion, be used as production units. Full-scale industrial bioreactors can range between 20 000 and 400 000 litres in volume. The management of scale-up requires high capital investment in mixing and aeration, in monitoring and control devices, and in stringent maintenance of sterility.

4.5   Media design for fermentation processes

Water is at the centre of all biotechnological processes and in most cases will be the dominant component of the media in which microorganisms will grow. After liquid fermentation processes have achieved optimum production, the removal of water is a major factor in the cost of bioproduct recovery and downstream processing. The quality of water is highly relevant as it affects microbial growth and the production of specific bioproducts. In the past, traditional brewing centres were established in localities where natural sources provided water of high quality without having to resort to extensive pre-treatment.

In media production there is usually quality control of the raw materials. It is increasingly being realised that, in respect of volume, water is one of the most important raw materials in many biotechnological processes and that its supply and use must be carefully monitored and controlled.

The basic nutritional requirements of microorganisms are an energy or carbon source, an available nitrogen source, inorganic elements and, for some

Table 4.8. Sources of carbohydrate and nitrogen for industrial media

Sources of carbohydrate	Sources of nitrogen (% nitrogen by weight)
Glucose	Barley (1.5–2.0)
Pure glucose monohydrate, hydrolysed starch	Beet molasses (1.5–2.0)
Lactose	Corn-steep liquor (4.5)
Pure lactose, whey powder	
Starch	Groundnut meal (8.0)
Barley, groundnut meal, oat flour, rye flour, soy	Oat flour (1.5–2.0)
bean meal	Pharmamedia (8.0)
Sucrose	Rye flour (1.5–2.0)
Beet molasses, cane molasses, crude brown sugar,	Soyabean meal (8.0)
pure white sugar	Whey powder (4.5)

cell types, specific growth factors. In most biotechnological processes carbon and nitrogen sources are more often derived from relatively complex mixtures of cheap natural products or by-products (Table 4.8).

Availability and type of nutrient can exert strong physiological control over fermentation reactors and product formation. Raw material input to a fermentation will be largely dependent on the cost of the material at a particular time since commodity market prices do alter with seasonal and other variables.

Sterilisation practices for biotechnological media must achieve maximum kill of contaminating microorganisms with minimum temperature damage to medium components. Mostly, batch-wise sterilisation in the bioreactor is still the most widely used method, although continuous methods are gaining increased acceptability.

Media preparation may seem to be a relatively uninteresting part of the overall bioprocess but it is in fact the cornerstone of the whole operation. Poor media design will lead to low efficiency of growth and concomitant poor product formation.

4.6   Solid-substrate fermentation

There are many biotechnological processes that involve the growth of microorganisms on solid substrates in the absence or near absence of free water (Table 4.9). The most regularly used solid substrates are cereal grains, legume seeds, wheat bran, lignocellulose materials such as straws, sawdust or wood

Table 4.9. Some examples of solid-substrate fermentations

Example	Substrate	Microorganism(s) involved
Mushroom production (European and Oriental)	Straw, manure	*Agaricus bisporus* *Lentinus edodes* *Volvariella volvacea*
Sauerkraut	Cabbage	Lactic acid bacteria
Soy sauce	Soya beans and wheat	*Aspergillus oryzae*
Tempeh	Soya beans	*Rhizopus oligosporus*
Ontjom	Peanut press cake	*Neurospora sitophila*
Cheeses	Milk curd	*Penicillium roquefortii*
Leaching of metals	Low-grade ores	*Thiobacillus* sp.
Organic acids	Cane sugar, molasses	*Aspergillus niger*
Enzymes	Wheat bran, etc.	*Aspergillus niger*
Composting	Mixed organic material	Fungi, bacteria, actinomycetes
Sewage treatment	Components of sewage	Bacteria, fungi and protozoa

shavings, and a wide range of plant and animal materials. Most of these compounds are invariably polymeric molecules – insoluble or sparingly soluble in water – but are mostly cheap and easily obtainable and represent a concentrated source of nutrients for microbial growth.

Many of these fermentations have great antiquity and, in many instances, there are records dating back hundreds of years. In the East, there is a wide array of food fermentations, including soy sauce and tempeh, as well as many large industrial enzyme processes. In the West, the fermentation processes have centred on the production of silage, mushroom cultivation, cheese and sauerkraut production, and the composting of plant and animal wastes. Solid-substrate fermentations using recyclable raw materials such as straw, wood and other waste materials could well be industries of the future, producing ethanol, methane and edible biomass.

The microbiological components of solid-substrate fermentations can occur as single pure cultures, mixed identifiable cultures or totally mixed indigenous microorganisms.

In many solid-substrate fermentations there is a need to pre-treat the substrate raw materials to enhance the availability of the bound nutrients and also to reduce the size of the components, e.g. pulverising straw and shredding vegetable materials in order to optimise the physical aspects of the process.

Table 4.10. Advantages and disadvantages of solid-substrate fermentations (compared with liquid fermentations)

Advantages	Disadvantages
Simple media with cheaper natural, rather than costly, fossil-derived components.	Processes limited mainly to moulds that tolerate low moisture levels.
Low moisture content of materials gives economy of bioreactor space, low liquid effluent treatment, less microbial contamination, often no need to sterilise, easier downstream processing.	Metabolic heat production in large-scale operation creates problems.
Aeration requirements can be met by simple gas diffusion or by aerating intermittently, rather than continuously.	Process monitoring, e.g. moisture levels, biomass, O_2 and CO_2 levels, is difficult to achieve accurately.
Yields of products can be high.	Bioreactor design not well developed.
Low energy expenditure compared with stirred tank bioreactors.	Product limitation. Slower growth rate of microorganisms.

However, cost aspects of pre-treatment must be balanced with eventual product value. Bioreactor designs for solid-substrate fermentations are inherently more simple than for liquid cultivations. They are classified into fermentations (a) without agitation, (b) with occasional agitation, and (c) with continuous agitation. The relative advantages and disadvantages of solid-substrate fermentations when compared with liquid fermentations are represented in Table 4.10.

4.7   Technology of mammalian and plant cell culture

The main impetus to achieve mass *in vitro* cultivation of mammalian cells dates from the early 1950s with the need to produce large quantities of polio vaccine. During the second half of the twentieth century there was a major drive to develop media and cultivation practices to produce viable and actively proliferating cell cultures from a wide range of different organisms – from mammals such as humans, rats, mice, hampsters, monkeys, cattle, sheep and horses, and, more recently, from fish and insects. Specific cell lines have been obtained from human organs such as the liver, kidney, lungs, lymph nodes, lung, heart and ovaries, together with an extensive range of various cancer cell lines.

In their natural environment, mammalian cells will obtain the necessary nutrients for metabolism and growth by way of blood circulation. To mimic the complexity of the blood supply has been a continuing area of study and now many successful media formulations have been achieved which will vary in make-up depending on the cell type. Most media will normally contain a complex mixture of organic compounds, such as amino acids, vitamins, organic acids and others, together with buffering inorganic salts. Some media still contain blood serum (5–20%) for the supply of growth factors, trace elements, lipids and other unknown factors. However, the use of serum creates many problems, including variability of nutrient content between batches, irregularity of supply, and now more recently the concern that serum may be contaminated with virions or prion particles.

When mammalian cells are cultured, they grow as unicellular organisms, multiplying by division provided that suitable nutrient and correct environmental conditions are available. Such cells differ from microbial and plant cells in lacking a rigid outer cell wall, making them vulnerable to shear forces and to changes in osmolarity. Furthermore, they are extremely sensitive to impurities in water, to the cost and quality control of media, and the need to avoid contamination by more rapidly growing microorganisms.

Freshly isolated cultures from mammalian systems are known as '*primary cultures*' until subcultured. At this stage they are usually heterogeneous, but still closely representative of the parent cell types and in the expression of tissue-specific properties. After several subcultures onto fresh media, the cell line will either die out or 'transform' to become a *continuous* or *immortalised cell line*. Such cell lines show many alterations from the primary cultures, including changes in cytomorphology, increased growth rate, increase in chromosome variation and increase in tumorigenicity. *In vitro* transformation is primarily the acquisition of an infinite lifespan.

Mammalian cells can be grown either in an unattached suspension culture or attached to a solid surface. Cells such as HeLa cells (cells derived from a human malignancy) can grow in either state, lymphoblastoid cells can grow in suspension culture, while primary or normal diploid cells will only grow when they are attached to a solid surface. Most future commercial development with mammalian cells will be dominated by the cultivation of anchorage-dependent cell types.

Monolayer cultivation of animal cells is governed by the surface area available for attachment, and design considerations have been directed to methods of increasing surface area. Early designs relied mainly on roller tubes or bottles to ensure the exchange of nutrients and gases. A recent sophisticated system supports the growth of cells in coils of gas-permeable Teflon tubing, each tube having a surface area of 10 000 cm^2; up to 20 such coils can be incorporated into an incubator chamber. A wide range of cells have been successfully cultured under these conditions.

Suspension cultures have been successfully developed to quite large bioreactor volumes, thus allowing all the engineering advantages of the stirred tank bioreactor, which have accrued from microbial studies, to be used to advantage. Such studies have only been on a batch-culture basis.

A combination of attachment culture and suspension culture by the use of microcarrier and porous microcarrier beads has been a major recent innovation in this area. In principle, the anchorage-dependent cells attach to special DEAE-Sephadex beads (having a surface area of 7 cm^2/mg), which are able to float in suspension. In this way the engineering advantages of the stirred tank bioreactor may be used with anchored cells. Many cell types have been grown in this manner, with successful production of viruses and human interferon. The undoubted success of the microcarrier beads may eventually lead to the demise of conventional monolayer systems. New bioreactor designs involving the microcarrier bead concept will surely create a wider commercial development of animal and human cell types.

While such cell lines have allowed extensive studies in mammalian cell biochemistry, the major practical applications have included: vaccine production (polio, mumps, rabies, etc.), toxicological and pharmaceutical research with the aim of reducing animal testing, the production of artificial organs and skin, and the extensive use of mammalian cell lines as producers of proteins for diagnostic (monoclonal antibodies) and for therapeutic applications (interferons, hormones, insulin, etc.). The introduction of foreign genes into mammalian cell lines is now relatively commonplace and will be relevant to improving cell lines in many ways, such as extending productivity, the ability to grow on serum-free media, and to increasing the range of productivity of human therapeutic molecules.

The use of plant cell culture techniques for the micropropagation of certain plants is discussed in Chapter 10. In such cases, plant cell cultures will progress through organogenesis, plantlet amplification and eventual establishment in soil. However, large-scale production of suspension cell cultures of many plant species has now been achieved and yields of products typical of the whole plant have been impressive, e.g. nicotine, alkaloids and ginseng. It is now envisaged that large-scale fermentation programmes may be able to produce commercially acceptable levels of certain high-value plant products, e.g. digitalis, jasmine, spearmint and codeine.

The fermentation methods used to cultivate plant cells in liquid-agitated culture have been largely derived from microbial techniques. Plant cell culture is much slower than with microorganisms, though most of the other characteristics of fermentation are quite similar. The volume of an average cultured plant cell can be up to 200 000 times that of a bacterial cell. Although some plant products are now appearing on the market, it is not expected to be commercially attractive for some time.

4.8   Downstream processing

Downstream processing refers to the isolation and purification of a biotechnologically formed product to a state suitable for the intended use. In most, but not all, biotechnology processes the desired product(s) will be in dilute aqueous solution and the ultimate level of downstream processing will mirror the type of product and required degree of purity. The range of products is considerable and varied in form and can include whole cells, amino acids, vitamins, organic acids, solvents, enzymes, vaccines, therapeutic proteins and monoclonal antibodies. Within these products there will be considerable variation in molecular size and chemical complexity, and a wide range of separation methods will be required for recovery and purification. While many of the products are relatively stable in structure, others can be highly labile and require careful application of the methodology.

The design and efficient operation of downstream processing operations are vital elements in getting the required products into commercial use and should reflect the need not to lose more of the desired product than is absolutely necessary. An example of the effort expended in downstream processing is provided by the plant Eli Lilly built to produce human insulin (Humulin). Over 90% of the 200 staff are involved in recovery processes. Thus, downstream processing of biotechnological processes represents a major part of the overall costs of most processes but is also the least-heralded aspect of biotechnology. Improvements in downstream processing will benefit the overall efficiency and costs of the processes.

Downstream processing will primarily be concerned with initial separation of the bioreactor broth into a liquid phase and a solids phase and subsequent concentration and purification of the product. Downstream processing is a multistage operation (Table 4.11). Methods in use or proposed range from conventional to the arcane, including distillation, centrifuging, filtration, ultrafiltration, solvent extraction, adsorption, selective membrane technology, reverse osmosis, molecular sieves, electrophoresis and affinity

Table 4.11. Downstream processing operations

Operation	Method
Separation	Filtration
	Centrifugation
	Flotation
	Disruption
Concentration	Solubilisation
	Extraction
	Thermal processing
	Membrane filtration
	Precipitation
Purification	Crystallisation
	Chromatography
Modification	
Drying	

chromatography. It is in this area that several potential industrial applications of modern biotechnology have come to grief either because the extraction has defeated the ingenuity of the designers or, more probably, because the extraction process has required so much energy input as to render it uneconomic.

Final products of the downstream purification stages should have some degree of stability for commercial distribution. Stability is best achieved for most products by using some form of drying. In practice, this is achieved by spray drying, fluidised-bed drying or by freeze drying. The method of choice is product- and cost-dependent. Products sold in the dry form include organic acids, amino acids, antibiotics, polysaccharides, enzymes, SCP and many others. Many products cannot be supplied easily in a dried form and must be sold in liquid preparations. Care must be taken to avoid microbial contamination and deterioration and, when the product is proteinaceous, to avoid denaturation.

The role of downstream processing will continue to be one of the most challenging and demanding parts of many biotechnological processes. Purity and stability are the hallmarks of most high-value biotechnological products.

It can be said that biotechnological processes will, in most part, need to be contained within a defined area or bioreactor and, to a large extent, the ultimate success of most of the processes will depend on the correct choice and operation of these systems. For most high-value products, cultivation of the producer organism will normally be by monoculture, requiring complete asepsis to maximise product formation. On the industrial side, the scale of operation will, for economic reasons, mainly be very large, and in almost all cases the final success will require the closest cooperation between the bioscientist, the chemist and the process or biochemical engineer – in this way demonstrating the truly interdisciplinary nature of biotechnological processes.

4.9   Postscript

It is now recognised that the production of microorganisms and their products for a multitude of purposes is now a worldwide activity. The know-how technology, equipment and materials are now routinely used for entirely legitimate, peaceful and creative purposes. Regrettably, they can also be used for the production of biological weapons. In biological warfare, specific microorganisms or derived toxins which can cause disease in humans, animals or plants or which harm the environment can be used to achieve military and/or political objectives. Furthermore, unlike nuclear and chemical weapons, biological weapons are relatively easy and cheap to produce and manufacture and can also be carried out on a small scale. Such sinister use of microbial biotechnology must be totally outlawed by world governments.

5

Enzyme technology

5.1 The nature of enzymes

Enzymes are complex organic molecules present in living cells where they act as catalysts in bringing about chemical changes in substances. With the development of the science of biochemistry has come a fuller understanding of the wide range of enzymes present in living cells and of their modes of action. Without enzymes, there can be no life. Although enzymes are only formed in living cells, many can be separated from the cells and can continue to function *in vitro*. This unique ability of enzymes to perform their specific chemical transformations in isolation has led to an ever-increasing use of enzymes in industrial and food processes, in bioremediation, and in medicine, and their production is collectively termed 'enzyme technology'.

The activity of an enzyme is due to its catalytic nature. An enzyme carries out its activity without being consumed in the reaction, and the reaction occurs at a very much higher rate when the enzyme is present. Enzymes are highly specific and function only on designated types of compounds – the substrates. A minute amount of enzyme can react with a large amount of substrate. The catalytic function of the enzyme is due not only to its primary molecular structure but also to the intricate folding configuration of the whole enzyme molecule. It is this configuration which endows the protein with its specific catalytic function; disturb the configuration by, for example, a change in pH or temperature, and the activity can be lost. For some enzymes there is an obligatory need for additional factors, termed 'co-factors', that can be metal ions, nucleotides, etc. Because of their specificity, enzymes can differentiate between chemicals with closely related structures and can catalyse

Table 5.1. Distribution of bulk-produced enzymes

Specific area	Percentage
Food	41
Detergents	34
Textiles	11
Leather	3
Pulp/paper	1
Other applications	6

reactions over a wide range of temperatures ($0–110°C$) and in the pH range 2–14. In industrial applications this can result in high-quality products, fewer by-products and simpler purification procedures. Furthermore, enzymes are non-toxic and biodegradable (an attractive 'green' issue) and can be produced especially from microorganisms in large amounts without the need for special chemical-resistant equipment.

Enzyme technology embraces production, isolation, purification and use in soluble or immobilised form. Commercially produced enzymes will undoubt-edly contribute to the solution of some of the most vital problems with which modern society is confronted, e.g. food production, energy shortage and preservation, and improvement of the environment, together with numer-ous medical applications. This new technology has its origins in biochemistry but has drawn heavily on microbiology, chemistry and process engineering to achieve the present status of the science. For the future, enzyme technology and genetic engineering will be two very closely related areas of study dealing with the application of genes and their products. Together, these sciences will attempt to exploit creatively the continuous flow of discoveries being made by molecular geneticists and enzymologists.

It is estimated that the world market for enzymes is over $2 billion and will double over the next decade. There are now over 400 companies world-wide involved in enzyme production, with European companies dominating (60%) and the USA and Japan with 55%. Bulk enzyme distribution in various industries is shown in Table 5.1 and production of specific bulk enzymes is shown in Table 5.2.

5.2   The application of enzymes

For thousands of years processes such as brewing, breadmaking and production of cheeses have involved the serendipitous use of enzymes (see Table 5.3). The

Table 5.2. Approximate annual world production of some industrial enzymes

Enzyme	Tonnes pure enzyme
Bacillus protease	550
Amyloglucosidase	350
Bacillus amylase	350
Glucose isomerase	60
Microbial rennet	25
Fungal amylase	20
Pectinase	20
Fungal protease	15

Greek epic poems the *Odyssey* and the *Iliad,* dating around 700 BC, both refer to the use of what we now recognise as enzymes in cheese making. In this way, traditional practices and technologies that relied on enzymic conversions were well established before any coherent body of knowledge on their rational application had been developed.

In the West, the industrial understanding of enzymes revolved around yeast and malt where traditional baking and brewing industries were rapidly expanding. Much of the early development of biochemistry was centred around yeast fermentations and processes for conversion of starch to sugar. In the East, the comparable industries were sake production and many food fermentations, all of which made use of bacteria and filamentous fungi as the sources of enzyme activity. The year 1896 saw the true beginnings of modern microbial enzyme technology with the first marketing in the West of takadiastase – a rather crude mixture of hydrolytic enzymes prepared by growing the fungus *Aspergillus oryzae* on wheat bran. The method of takadiastase production varied little from that practised for thousands of years in Asia, but it did represent an important transfer of technology from East to West.

Leather has always been an important commodity and, originally, the process by which hides were softened before tanning – termed 'bating' – was most obnoxious, requiring the use of dog faeces and pigeon droppings. However, at the turn of this century, Otto Rohm, a distinguished German chemist, determined that the active components in dog faeces were proteases – enzymes which degrade proteins. He was able to demonstrate that extracts from animal organs which produced similar enzymes could be used instead of the faeces and, from 1905, pig and cow pancreases were to provide a more socially acceptable and reliable source of these enzymes.

Table 5.3. Industrial applications of enzymes

Application	Enzymes used	Uses	Problems
Biological detergents	Primarily proteinases, produced in an extracellular form from bacteria	Used for pre-soak conditions and direct liquid applications	Allergic response of process workers; now overcome by encapsulation techniques
	Amylase enzymes	Detergents for machine dishwashing to remove resistant starch residues	
Baking industry	Fungal α-amylase enzymes; normally inactivated about 50°C; destroyed during baking process	Catalyse breakdown of starch in the flour to sugar, which can be used by the yeast. Used in production of white bread, buns and rolls.	
	Proteinase enzymes	Biscuit manufacture to lower the protein level of the flour	
Brewing industry	Enzymes produced from barley during mashing stage of beer production	Degrade starch and proteins to produce simple sugars, amino acids and peptides – used by the yeasts to enhance alcohol production.	
	Industrially produced enzymes: amylases, glucanases, proteinases β-glucanase amyloglucosidase proteinases	Now widely used in the brewing process: split polysaccharides and proteins in the malt improve filtration characteristics low-calorie beer remove cloudiness during storage of beers	

(cont.)

Table 5.3. (cont.)

Application	Enzymes used	Uses	Problems
Dairy industry	Rennin, derived from the stomachs of young ruminant animals (calves, lambs, kids)	Manufacture of cheese, used to split protein	Older animals cannot be used as, with increasing age, rennin production decreases and is replaced by another proteinase, pepsin, which is not suitable for cheese production. In recent years the great increase in cheese consumption together with increased beef production have resulted in increasing shortage of rennin and escalating prices.
	Microbially produced enzyme	Now finding increasing use in the dairy industry	
	Lipases	Enhance ripening of blue-mould cheeses (Danish Blue, Roquefort)	
	Lactases	Break down lactose to glucose and galactose	
Starch industry	Amylases, amyloglucosidases and glucoamylases	Convert starch into glucose and various syrups	
	Glucose isomerase	Converts glucose into fructose (high-fructose syrups derived from starchy materials have enhanced sweetening properties and lower calorific values)	
	Immobilised enzymes	Production of high-fructose syrups	Widely used in the USA and Japan but EEC restrictive practices to protect sugar-beet farmers prohibit use.

Industry / use	Enzyme	Description	
Textile industry	Amylase enzymes	Now widely used to remove starch which is used as an adhesive, or size, on threads of certain fabrics to prevent damage during weaving. (Traditionally, desizing using strong chemicals has prevailed.)	
	Bacterial enzymes	Generally preferred for desizing since they are able to withstand working temperatures of up to 100–110°C.	
Leather industry	Enzymes found in dog and pigeon dung	Traditionally used to treat leather to make it pliable by removing certain protein components. (The process is called 'bating'; strong bating required to achieve a soft, pliable leather, slight bating for the soles of shoes.)	Offensive preparation
	Trypsin enzymes from slaughterhouses and from microorganisms	Now largely replacing the enzymes mentioned above for bating. Also used for removing the hair from hides and skins.	
Medical and pharmaceutical uses	Trypsin	Débridement of wounds, dissolving blood clots	
	Pancreatic trypsin	Digestive aid formulations, treatment of inflammations, etc.	
		Many enzymes used in clinical chemistry as diagnostic tools	

The early local use of enzymes in various processes relied on plant and animal sources. Proteases such as papain from papaya, ficin from figs and bromelain from pineapple are still important commercial sources. From animals, there are still considerable viable sources for esterases, proteases and lipases such as rennets, pepsin, chymosin and lysozyme. While these sources of enzymes continue to have industrial importance, they do have limitations, including lack of consistent quality and availability and, in the case of some plant enzymes, disturbance of supply due to weather and political instability at source.

It was not until the mid-1950s that rapid development in enzyme technology occurred, using, in particular, microbial enzyme sources. The reasons for this are varied but depended largely on the following:

(1) There was a major development in submerged cultivation practices, with microorganisms primarily associated with the World War II penicillin production processes, and this newly acquired knowledge was readily applied to the large-scale cultivation of other microorganisms and subsequently for microbial enzyme production.
(2) Basic knowledge of enzyme properties was rapidly expanding and this led to the realisation of the potential for using enzymes as industrial catalysts.
(3) Most enzymes of potential industrial importance could be produced from some microorganism.

The further development of enzymes as additives was largely to provide enhancement of traditional processes rather than to open up new possibilities. Even now, most bulk production of crude enzymes is concerned largely with enzymes that hydrolyse the glucosidic links of carbohydrates such as starch and pectins and with the proteases that hydrolyse the peptide links of proteins.

Approximately 90% of bulk enzyme production is derived from microorganisms such as filamentous fungi, bacteria and yeasts, and the remainder from animals (6%) and plants (4%).

Cell-free enzymes have many advantages over chemical processes where a number of sequential reactions are involved. In fermentation processes the use of microbial cells as catalysts can have a number of limitations:

(1) A high proportion of the substrate will normally be converted to biomass;
(2) Wasteful side reactions may occur;
(3) The conditions for growth of the microorganisms may not be the same as for product formation;
(4) The isolation and purification of the desired product from the fermentation liquor may be difficult.

Many, if not all, of these limitations may be alleviated by the use of purified enzymes and possibly by the further use of enzymes in an immobilised form. In the future many traditional fermentations may be replaced by multi-enzyme reactors that would create highly efficient rates of substrate utilisation, higher yields and higher product uniformity.

There is now a rapid proliferation of uses and potential uses for more highly purified enzyme preparations in industrial processing, clinical medicine and laboratory practice. The range of pure enzymes now available commercially is rapidly increasing. Enzymes that are sold at over 10 000 tonnes annually cost US$5–30 per kilogram, and speciality enzymes of less than 1 tonne cost US$50 000 per kilogram, while therapeutic enzymes can cost over US$5000 per gram.

In many operations, such as clarifying wines and juices, chill proofing of beer and improving bread doughs, the use of crude enzymes is likely to add very little to the cost of the product. Most of the enzymes used on an industrial scale are extracellular enzymes, i.e. enzymes that are normally excreted by the microorganism to act upon their substrate in an external environment, and are analogous to the digestive enzymes of man and animals. Thus, when microorganisms produce enzymes to split large external molecules into an assimilable form, the enzymes are usually excreted into the fermentation media. In this way the fermentation broth from the cultivation of certain microorganisms, e.g. bacteria, yeasts or filamentous fungi, then becomes a major source of proteases, amylases and (to a lesser extent) cellulases, lipases, etc. Most industrial enzymes are hydrolases and are capable of acting without complex co-factors; they are readily separated from microorganisms without rupturing the cell walls, and are water soluble.

Some intracellular enzymes are now being produced industrially and include glucose oxidase for food preservation, asparaginase for cancer therapy and penicillin acylase for antibiotic conversion. Since most cellular enzymes are, by nature, intracellular, more advances can be expected in this area.

The sales of industrial enzymes were relatively small up until about 1965 (Fig. 5.1), when enzymes in detergents came into general use. There was a massive increase in the use of enzymes in detergents between 1966 and 1969, but this was to collapse between 1969 and 1970, when apparent allergic symptoms were discovered in workers handling enzymes at the factory level. There was much press hysteria and enzymes were mostly taken out of detergents. However, with proper precautions in the factories and by encapsulating the enzymes before reaching the customer, the postulated risks were eliminated; careful studies found no adverse environmental effects from the use of enzymes nor any effects on domestic users. Once again, the application of enzymes in

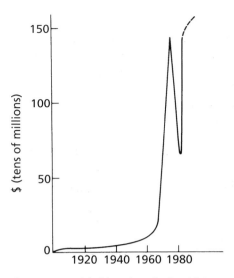

Fig. 5.1 Worldwide sales of microbial enzymes.

detergents has achieved good levels, and there is a steady growth in the use of enzymes in that part of the detergent industry where enzymes can improve washing results.

In western Europe, hot water washes (approx. 65–70°C) have been considered essential for most clothes cleaning operations, whereas in the USA and Canada most machines operate at 55°C. In complete contrast, in Japan clothes are usually washed for longer periods with cold water. Thus, universally there is increased interest in the use of detergent enzymes that function well at relatively low temperatures, i.e. 20–30°C. While proteases have dominated the detergent market, there is increasing use of amylases and lipases for the removal of starches and fats. Cellulase has recently entered the detergent market and, unlike the other enzymes which degrade particular stains, the cellulases act directly on the fabric. When new, cotton consists of smooth fibres, but with prolonged use and washing, microfibrils or broken strands of fibre create a 'fuzz' or roughness on the fabric surface. The cellulases remove this and so improve the appearance and feel or smoothness of the fabric. Cellulases are also used to restore the colour of cotton that has been washed several times and to give jeans the so-called 'stone-wash' look.

In the starch industry, α-amylase and amyloglucosidase have substituted for acid completely in the manufacture of dextrose, and with other enzymes in the production of vitamin C, amino acids, antibiotics and steroids.

Enzyme prices have fallen in real terms over the past decade. For example, the bulk quantities of enzymes for most food applications are now, at least in relative terms, 20–35% cheaper than in the mid-1970s. More specialised enzymes, used in smaller concentrations and in higher purities, have increased in use on account of improved production methods. Further large-scale uses of enzymes as catalysts will be achieved only if their costs continue to fall. Current sales of industrial enzymes worldwide are between $650 and $750 million according to the US Department of Commerce. In financial terms, 80% of the industrial enzyme sales goes to three principal markets: starch conversion (40%), detergents (30%) and dairy applications, particularly rennets (10%). Animal rennet sales for cheese manufacturing are approaching $100 million and animal rennet is being strongly augmented by microbial and genetically engineered rennets. However, the growth of enzyme sales has been, and continues to be, heavily influenced by the starch and detergent industries. Innovations such as recombinant DNA technologies and improved fermentation methods and downstream processing will increasingly reduce production costs, particularly of high-cost enzymes, making them more competitive with other chemical processes.

Although many specific enzymes are being increasingly used in clinical or diagnostic applications, the amount of enzymes actually needed is quite small. This arises from the development of automated procedures which use immobilised enzymes and seek to miniaturise the system, with the enzyme becoming analogous to the microchip in a computer. Thus, although the enzyme is essential, the market need is quite small.

When enzymes are used as bulk additives, only 1 or 2 kilograms will normally be required to react with 1000 kilograms of substrate. In this way, the cost of the enzyme will be US$3–25 per kilogram or 10–14% of the value of the end-product. Such enzymes are usually sold in liquid formulations and are rarely purified. In contrast, diagnostic enzymes will generally be used in milligram or microgram quantities and can cost up to US$100 000 per kilogram. Such enzymes will be required in a high state of purity.

The further growth of world enzyme markets will revolve around: (a) high-volume, industrial-grade enzyme products, and (b) low-volume, high-purity enzyme products for analytical, diagnostic or therapeutic applications. In the world production of industrial enzymes it is of interest that two small European countries (Holland and Denmark) dominate the markets (Table 5.4).

Among the many new areas of opportunity for enzyme technology is the utilisation of *lignocellulose* (or woody materials) in biotechnological processes. This abundant substrate must be utilised, and many research efforts are now being directed to discover new and efficient enzyme systems that can attack the complex molecular configurations of lignocellulose and make available the component molecules. This could well be the most bountiful future area of expansion in enzyme technology.

Table 5.4. Production of industrial enzymes by tonnage in the western world

Nation	Enzyme production (tonnes)	%
USA	6 360	12
Japan	4 240	8
Denmark	24 910	47
France	1 590	3
Germany (West)	3 180	6
Netherlands	10 070	19
UK	1 060	2
EU	40 810	77
Switzerland	1 060	2
Others	530	1
Total	53 000	100

5.3   Genetic engineering and protein engineering of enzymes

Recombinant DNA technology has allowed the transfer of useful enzyme-genes from one organism to another. Thus, when a good candidate enzyme for industrial use has been identified, the relevant gene can be cloned into a more suitable production host microorganism (Fig. 5.2) and an industrial fermentation carried out. In this way it becomes possible to produce industrial enzymes of very high quantity and purity.

Recombinant microorganisms are now becoming a dominant source of a wide variety of types of enzymes. This trend will increase in the future owing to the ease of genetic engineering and the almost unlimited variety of enzymes available from microorganisms in diverse and extreme environments, from fastidious microorganisms and from others that are potential pathogens. Enzymes from extremophyles, such as microorganisms that are able to grow at high temperatures (90–100°C), can now be grown in mesophyllic microorganisms and produce enzymes which have high temperature resistance and which can be used in industrial processes.

A recent example of this technology is the detergent enzyme Lipolase, produced by Novo Nordisk A/S, which has improved removal of fat stains in fabrics. The enzyme was first identified in the fungus *Humicola lanuginosa*

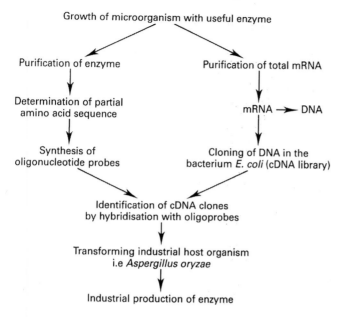

Fig. 5.2   Cloning strategy for enzymes.

at levels that were inappropriate for commercial production. The gene DNA fragment for the enzyme was cloned into the production fungus *Aspergillus oryzae* and commercial levels of enzyme achieved. The enzyme has proved efficient under many wash conditions. The enzyme is also very stable at a variety of temperatures and pH conditions relevant to washing. Furthermore, Lipolase is remarkably resistant to proteolytic activity of the commonly used detergent proteases.

The modification of enzymes to improve/alter their catalytic properties has been carried out for several decades. In the past, this was achieved by random multinational programmes, but in recent years advanced technology has brought about major changes in the field. Table 5.5 gives some of the main objectives to which this research has been directed.

Protein engineering or 'molecular surgery' has been used to alter the performance of enzyme molecules. Protein engineering of enzymes involves the creation of a three-dimensional graphical model of the purified enzyme obtained from X-ray crystallographic data. Changes to the enzyme structure can then be considered which might result in increased stability to, for example, pH and temperature and the requisite molecular changes made in the gene coding for the enzyme.

Table 5.5. Objectives for the preparation of modified enzymes

(1) To enhance the activity of the enzyme
(2) To improve the stability
(3) To permit the enzyme to function in a changed environment
(4) To change pH or temperature optima
(5) To change the specificity of an enzyme so that it catalyses the conversion of a different substrate
(6) To change the reaction catalysed
(7) To enhance the efficiency of a process

Adapted from Gray (1990).

Two main avenues of research have been pursued in order to alter the performance of enzymes. In one approach, mutagenesis of the cloned-gene product – amino acid residues at defined positions in the structure of the enzyme – can be replaced by other suitably coded amino acid residues. The altered gene is then transformed into a suitable host organism and the mutant enzyme subsequently produced with the requisite changes in position. This process is known as 'site-directed mutagenesis'. The second method used involves the isolation of the natural enzyme and modifications to its structure carried out by chemical or enzymatic means – sometimes referred to as 'chemical' mutation. A successful example of protein engineering is that of the enzyme phospholipase A2, which was modified structurally to resist higher concentrations of acid. This enzyme is widely used as a food emulsifier.

Clearly, genetic engineering and protein engineering will have dramatic impacts on the enzyme industry in its many forms. Genetic engineering will ensure better product economy, production of enzymes from rare microorganisms, faster development programmes, etc. Also, extensive tests of the enzymes now used have shown no harmful effects on the environment.

5.4 The technology of enzyme production

Although many useful enzymes have been derived from plant and animal sources, it is clear that most future developments in enzyme technology will rely on enzymes of microbial origin. Even in the malting process of brewing, where the amylases of germinated barley which hydrolyse the starch are relatively inexpensive and around which existing brewing technology has developed, there are now some competitive processes involving microbial enzymes.

The use of microorganisms as a source material for enzyme production has developed for several important reasons:

(1) There is normally a high specific activity per unit dry weight of product.
(2) Seasonal fluctuations of raw materials and possible shortages due to climatic change or political upheavals do not occur.
(3) In microbes, a wide spectrum of enzyme characteristics, such as pH range and high temperature resistance, is available for selection.
(4) Industrial genetics has greatly increased the possibilities for optimising enzyme yield and type through strain selection, mutation, induction and selection of growth conditions and, more recently, by using the innovative powers of gene transfer technology and protein engineering.

Novel enzymes from unusual sources can now be produced by cloning the relevant gene into a well-characterised and easily grown microorganism such as *Aspergilus oryzae*.

The rationale for selection between different microorganisms is complex and involves many ill-defined factors such as economics of cultivation, whether the enzyme is secreted in the culture broth or retained in the cell, and the presence of harmful enzymes. Depending on source material, enzymes differ greatly in their stability to temperature and to extremes of pH. Thus, *Bacillus subtilis* proteases are relatively heat-stable and active under alkaline conditions and have been most suitable as soap-powder additives. In contrast, fungal amylases, because of their greater sensitivity to heat, have been more useful in the baking industry.

When selecting for enzyme production, the industrial geneticist must seek to optimise desired properties (high enzyme yield, stability, independence of inducers, good recovery, etc.) while also attempting to remove or suppress undesirable properties (harmful accompanying metabolites, odour, colour, etc.). Sophisticated genetic techniques have not yet been widely practised, most manufacturers relying mainly on mutagenisation combined with good selection methods. A common feature of most industrial producer organisms is that their genetics is little understood. However, gene transfer technology, together with protein engineering, will alter this and present new horizons to enzyme technology.

The raw materials for industrial enzyme fermentations have normally been limited to substances which are readily available in large quantities at low cost, and which are nutritionally safe. Some of the most commonly used substrates are starch hydrolysate, molasses, corn-steep liquor, whey and many cereals.

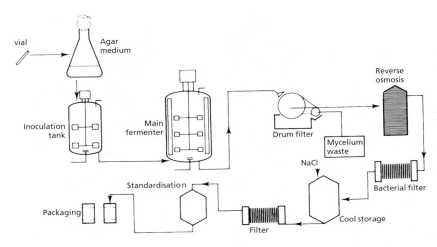

Fig. 5.3   The stages in the production of a liquid enzyme preparation.

Industrial enzyme production from microorganisms relies predominantly on either submerged liquid conditions or solid-substrate fermentation, as described in Chapter 4.

Solid-substrate methods of producing fungal enzymes have long historical applications, particularly in Japan and other Far East countries. In practice, this method uses moist wheat or rice bran with added nutrient salts as substrates. The growing environment is usually rectangular or circular trays held in constant-temperature rooms. Commercial enzymes of importance produced in this way include fungal amylases, proteases, pectinases and cellulases.

Since microbial enzymes are mostly low-volume, medium-cost products, the production methods using submerged liquid systems have generally relied on bioreactors that are similar in design and function to those used in antibiotic production processes (Fig. 5.3). The choice of fermentation medium is important since it supplies the energy needs as well as carbon and nitrogen sources. Raw material costs will be related closely to the value of the final product.

Enzyme synthesis in microorganisms is often repressed, i.e. the enzyme will only be produced in the presence of an inducer molecule – most often the substrate. The inducer functions by interfering with the controlling repressor, as exemplified by starch for amylase production and sucrose for invertase production. Feedback repression can occur in the biosynthesis of small molecules in which usually the first enzyme in the chain of production is inhibited by the final product. In some cases excess of specific nutrients, such as carbon,

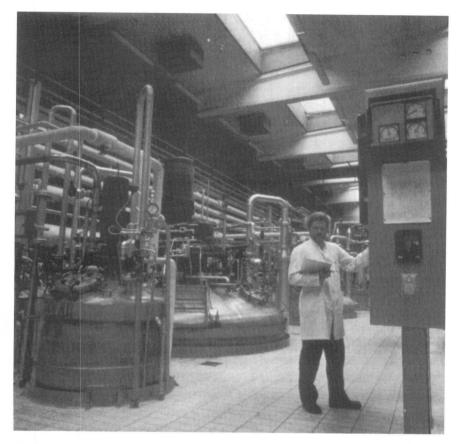

Fig. 5.4 Fermentation plant at Novo, Denmark, used for the production of enzyme.

nitrogen, etc., can shut down or repress the production of enzymes involved in related or unrelated compounds – catabolic repression.

The use of inducers for industrial enzyme production can often be difficult and the most common solution is to produce regulatory mutants in which inducer dependence has been eliminated by creating constituent mutants. For catabolic repression, mutants resistant to this phenomenon have been developed while it is also possible to control the effect of these substrates by feeding them into the bioreactor by a fed-batch regime.

A typical enzyme-producing bioreactor is constructed from stainless steel and has a capacity of 10–50 m^3 (Fig. 5.4). In most cases enzymes are produced in batch fermentations lasting from 30 to 150 hours; continuous-cultivation

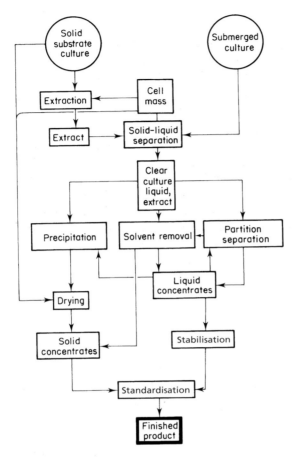

Fig. 5.5 The extraction and preparation of an enzyme

processes have found little application in industrial enzyme production. Sterility of the bioreactor system is essential throughout production.

At the completion of the fermentation, the enzyme may be present within the microorganism or excreted into the liquid or solid medium. Commercial enzyme preparations for sale will be either in a solid or a liquid form, crude or highly purified. The concentration and purification of an enzyme is shown in Fig. 5.5. Enzyme recovery and purification are as relevant to the economics of production as the fermentation stage. Enzyme purification will be carried out only if the extra cost is justified by the intended application of the enzyme. The scale of the purification or downstream processing will dictate the choice of separation techniques as some are difficult to operate on a large scale.

All microbial enzyme products that will be used in foods or medically related aspects are required to meet strict specifications with regard to toxicity (Table 5.6). At present, only a small number of microorganisms are used for enzyme production. Responsibility for the safety of an enzyme product remains with the manufacturer. In practice, a safe enzyme product should have low allergenic potential and be free of toxic materials and harmful microorganisms. Enzymes from animal and plant sources do not require toxicological studies to be performed. When enzymes are derived from microorganisms that are traditionally used in food or food processing, no testing is required (Table 5.6). Enzymes from other microorganisms may require extensive testing and also analysis for toxic metabolites such as exo- and endotoxins and mycotoxins. All bulk enzymes are supplied with a detailed Material Safety Data Sheet which covers potential dangers and also handling procedures for using the enzyme.

5.5   Immobilised enzymes

Almost 95% of all commercial enzymes are purchased in a soluble form, with the majority being used directly on a single-use basis in the areas listed in Table 5.1. The use of enzymes in a soluble or free form must be considered as very wasteful because the enzyme generally cannot be recovered at the end of the reaction. A new and valuable area of enzyme technology is that concerned with the immobilisation of enzymes on insoluble polymers, such as membranes and particles, which act as supports or carriers for the enzyme activity. The enzymes are physically confined during a continuous catalytic process and may be recovered from the reaction mixture and re-used over and over again, thus improving the economy of the process; this is merely a return to the natural immobilised state of most enzymes in living systems. Some enzymes that are rapidly inactivated by heat when in cell-free form can be stabilised by attachment to inert polymeric supports, while in other examples such insolubilised enzymes can be used in non-aqueous environments. Whole microbial cells can also be immobilised inside polyacrylamide beads and used for a wide range of catalytic functions. The variety of new enzymes and whole-organism systems that are likely to become cheaply available presents exciting possibilities for the future, especially in the pharmaceutical and diagnostic fields.

Table 5.6. Safety testing of food enzymes based on the Association of Microbial Food Enzyme Producers' classification

Group	(a) Microorganisms that have traditionally been used in food, or in food processing	(b) Microorganisms that are accepted as harmless contaminants present in food	(c) Microorganisms that are not included in either (a) or (b)
Test			
Pathogenicity	In general, no testing required		X
Acute oral toxicity, mouse and rat; subacute oral toxicity		X	X
Three-month oral toxicity, rat		X	X
In vitro mutagenicity		X	X
Teratogenicity, rat			X[a]
In vivo mutagenicity, mouse and hamster			X[a]
Toxicity studies on the final food			X[a]
Carcinogenicity, rat			X[a]
Fertility and reproduction			X[a]

X, test to be performed.
[a] Only to be performed under exceptional conditions.
From Godfrey and Reichelt (1983).

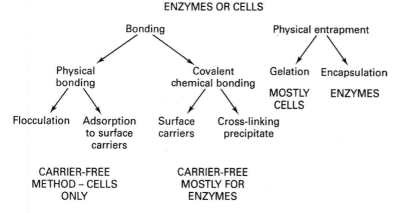

Fig. 5.6 Techniques of enzyme / cell immobilisation.

Present applications of immobilised catalysts are mainly confined to industrial processes, e.g. production of L-amino acids, organic acids and fructose syrup. The future potential for immobilised biocatalysts lies in novel applications and the development of new products rather than as an alternative to existing processes using non-immobilised biocatalysts.

Immobilised enzymes are normally more stable than their soluble counterparts and are able to be re-used in the purified semi-purified or whole-cell form. Catalytic properties of immobilised enzymes can often be altered favourably to allow operation under broader or more rigorous reaction conditions; for example, immobilised glucose isomerase can be used continuously for over 1000 hours at temperatures of 60–65°C.

How are enzymes immobilised? In practice, both physical and chemical methods are routinely used for enzyme immobilisation. Physically, enzymes may be absorbed onto an insoluble matrix, entrapped within a gel, or encapsulated within a microcapsule or behind a semi-permeable membrane (Fig. 5.6). Chemically, enzymes may be covalently attached to solid supports or cross linked.

A large number of chemical reactions have been used for the covalent binding of enzymes, by way of their non-essential functional groups, to inorganic carriers such as ceramics, glass, iron, zirconium and titanium, to natural polymers such as sepharose and cellulose, and to synthetic polymers such as nylon, polyacrylamide and other vinyl polymers and co-polymers possessing reactive chemical groups. In many of these procedures the covalent binding of enzymes to the carriers is non-specific, i.e. the binding of the enzyme to the carrier by way of the enzyme's chemically active groups distributed at random. More

Table 5.7. Limitations of immobilised enzyme techniques

Method	Advantages	Disadvantages
Covalent attachment	Not affected by pH, ionic strength of the medium or substrate concentration.	Active site may be modified; costly process.
Covalent crosslinking	Enzyme strongly bound, thus unlikely to be lost.	Loss of enzyme activity during preparation; not effective for macromolecular substrates; regeneration of carrier not possible.
Adsorption	Simple with no modification of enzyme; regeneration of carrier possible; cheap technique.	Changes in ionic strength may cause desorption; enzyme subject to microbial or proteolytic enzyme attack.
Entrapment	No chemical modification of enzyme.	Diffusion of substrate to, and product from, the active site; preparation difficult and often results in enzyme inactivation; continuous loss of enzyme due to distribution of pore size; not effective for macromolecular substrates; enzyme not subject to microbial or proteolytic action.

recent studies have attempted to develop techniques of enzyme immobilisation in which the enzyme binds to a carrier with high activity without affecting its catalytic activity. The limitations of immobilised enzyme techniques are shown in Table 5.7.

The entrapment of enzymes in gel matrices is achieved by carrying out the polymerisation or precipitation/coagulation reactions in the presence of the enzyme. Polyacrylamides, collagen, silica gel, etc., have all proved to be suitable matrices, but the entrapment process is relatively difficult and results in low enzyme activity.

Immobilised whole microbial cells are becoming increasingly utilised and tend to eliminate the tedious, time-consuming and expensive enzyme-purification steps. Immobilisation of whole cells is normally achieved by the

Table 5.8. The advantages of immobilised biocatalysts

(1) Permits the re-use of the component enzyme(s)
(2) Ideal for continuous operation
(3) Product is enzyme-free
(4) Permits more accurate control of catalytic processes
(5) Improves stability of enzymes
(6) Allows development of a multi-enzyme reaction system
(7) Offers considerable potential in industrial and medical use
(8) Reduces effluent disposal problems

same methods as for cell-free enzymes. The greatest potential for immobilised cell systems lies in replacing complex fermentations such as secondary product formation (i.e. semi-synthetic antibiotics) in the continuous monitoring of chemical processes (via enzyme electrodes), water analysis and waste treatment, continuous malting processes, nitrogen fixation, synthesis of steroids and other valuable medical products. The advantages of using immobilised biocatalysts are summarised in Table 5.8.

As a consequence of successful immobilisation techniques, in the form of enzyme capsules, enzyme beads, enzyme columns and enzyme membranes, many types of bioreactors have been developed on a laboratory scale and, to a lesser extent, on an industrial scale. These include *batch-stirred tank* bioreactors, continuous *packed-bed* bioreactors and continuous *fluidised-bed* bioreactors (Fig. 5.7). In industrial practice the catalytic properties of isolated enzymes, immobilised enzymes or immobilised whole cells are generally utilised within the confines of bioreactor vessels. Bioreactor systems can have many forms, depending on the type of reactions and stability of the enzyme.

In Europe, immobilised penicillin acylase is used to prepare 6-amino-penicillic acid (6-APA) from naturally produced penicillin G or V (Fig. 5.8). This compound is an important intermediate in the synthesis of semi-synthetic penicillins, which are so essential in our fight against bacterial diseases. Two types of penicillins are produced by industrial fermentation: penicillin G (phenyl acetyl-6-APA) and penicillin V (phenoxy acetyl-6-APA), each containing a nucleus of 6-APA and a side-chain. The antibiotic activity of the penicillin molecule is governed by the side-chain and, when removed and replaced with another, it can profoundly alter the antibiotic spectrum and other properties. Many pharmaceutical companies now operate immobilised enzyme processes for the production of 6-APA on an industrial scale.

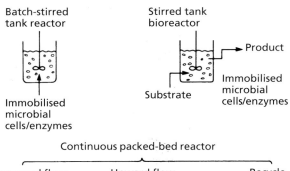

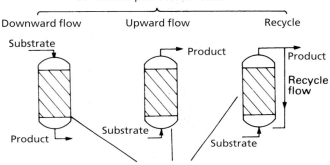

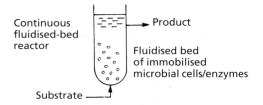

Fig. 5.7   Immobilised cell / enzyme bioreactors.

R–COHN $\xrightarrow{H_2O}$ H_2N + R–COOH

Penicillin acylase

Penicillin G or V   6-APA

Fig. 5.8   Formation of 6-APA by hydrolysis of penicillin.

Table 5.9. Some industrial applications of immobilised enzymes

Industry	Enzyme	Method of immobilisation	Process
Food	Glucose isomerase	AE-cellulose	Conversion of glucose to fructose
		Cell homogenates cross-linked with glutaraldehyde DEAE-Sephadex	
	Aminoacylase		Resolution of DL-amino acids to L-forin
Dairy	Lactase	Cellulose acetate fibres	Hydrolysis of lactose to glucose and galactose
Pharmaceutical	Penicillin G/V acylases	Br CN-activated Sephadex	Production of 6-APA from penicillin G
		Cellulose triacetate fibres Polyacrylamide	
Chemical	Nitrilase	Polyacrylamide	Production of acrylamide from acrylonitrile

At least 3500 tonnes of 6-APA are produced each year, requiring the production of about 30 tonnes of the enzyme (Table 5.9).

Immobilised glucose isomerase is used in the USA, Japan and Europe for the industrial production of high-fructose syrups by partial isomerisation of glucose derived from starch. Thousands of tonnes of high-fructose syrup are produced annually by this enzyme process, and it is undoubtedly the most widely used of all the immobilised enzymes. The industrial and commercial success of this process is due to the following facts: glucose derived from starch is relatively cheap; fructose is sweeter than glucose; the high-fructose syrup contains approximately equivalent amounts of glucose and fructose, and, from a nutritional aspect, is similar to sucrose. The overall production of fructose from starch is shown in Fig. 5.9.

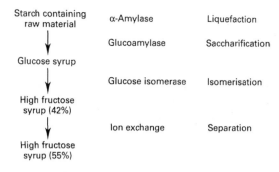

Fig. 5.9 Production of fructose from starch.

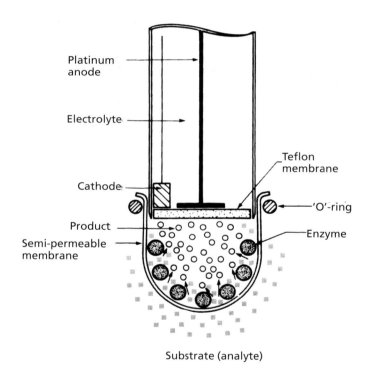

Fig. 5.10 A simple biosensor combining an electrochemical electrode and an enzyme immobilised onto a semi-permeable membrane (from Wymer, NCBE Newsletter).

Another important use of immobilised enzymes is aminoacylase production of amino acids. Aminoacylase columns are used in Japan to produce thousands of kilograms of L-methionine, L-phenylalanine, L-tryptophan and L-valine.

Enzyme polymer conjugates are now being used extensively in analytical and clinical chemistry. Immobilised enzyme columns or tubes can be used repeatedly as specific catalysts in assays of substrates. *Enzyme electrodes* are a new type of detector or biosensor designed for the potentiometric or amperometric assay of substrates such as urea, amino acids, glucose, alcohol and lactic acid. In design, the electrode is composed of a given electrochemical sensor in close contact with a thin, permeable enzyme membrane that is capable of reacting specifically with the given substrates. The embedded enzymes in the membrane produce O_2, hydrogen ions, ammonium ions, CO_2 or other small molecules, depending on the enzymatic reactions occurring, which are readily detected by the specific sensor; the magnitude of the response determines the concentration of the substrate (Fig. 5.10). While the biological component in a biosensor may more often be an enzyme or multi-enzyme system, it can also be an antibody, an organelle, a microbial cell or whole slices of tissue.

The application of enzyme technology to existing processes, e.g. brewing, food processing, medicine, pharmaceuticals, chemical industry and waste treatment, has enormous potential and is examined in later chapters.

Looking to the future, it seems reasonable to expect that the production and application of enzymes will continue to expand. The growing world concern about the environment and natural resources, in particular the rising prices of oil and other raw materials, is promoting new avenues of research and there is little doubt that enzymes will play a major role in solving some of these problems.

6

Biological fuel generation

As world populations continue to increase, there is also a growing *per capita* demand for energy. Coupled to this are the international commitments to reduce carbon dioxide emissions that were agreed at the Kyoto Conference.

6.1 Photosynthesis: the ultimate energy resource

The total economically recoverable world reserves of the three main fossil fuels, namely coal, natural gas and oil – applying current technology and assuming continued consumption of present-day rates – are, respectively, less than 1000 years, 35 years and 16 years. Modern industry is almost totally dependent on these limited supplies. Approximately 93% of fossil fuel consumed throughout the world is for energy production, with only 7% being used by industry for the production of solvents, plastics and a host of other organic chemicals.

The continual depletion of global fossil-fuel energy has generated an ever-increasing need to seek out alternative sources of energy. These have so far included: the harnessing of hydro-, tidal, wave and wind power; the capture of solar and geothermal energy supplies; and the much misunderstood, but most significant – nuclear power. With all of these systems there is as yet no definitive answer on both the economic and energetic outlay necessary for successful operation. However, it cannot be doubted that fossil fuels *will* disappear completely in the not too distant future.

There is now a growing appreciation of biological energy systems and that biotechnological advances in this area may soon bring economic reality to selected processes. Biomass such as forest, agricultural and animal residues, and industrial and domestic organic wastes, can now be converted by physico-chemical and/or fermentation processes to clean fuels and petrochemical substitutes. As fossil-fuel resources are depleted and become increasingly expensive, the conversion of organic residues to liquid fuels becomes a more economically attractive consideration. Photosynthetically derived material is not generally in a sufficiently dry state to possess an attractive calorific value, nor in a form that is best suited to modern technology.

Photosynthetic organisms, both terrestrial and marine, can be considered as continuous solar energy converters and are constantly renewable. Plant photosynthesis alone fixes about 2×10^{11} tonnes of carbon with an energy content of 2×10^{21} joules, which represents about 10 times the world's annual energy use and 200 times our food energy consumption. The magnitude and role of photosynthesis has gone largely unappreciated because we use such a small proportion of the fixed carbon. Let it not be forgotten that photosynthesis in the past provided all the present fossil carbon sources, namely coal, oil and natural gas. Thus, photosynthetically derived biomass that exists in many available forms in the environment could well be transformed into storable fuels and chemical feedstocks, such as alcohols and methane gas. The actual efficiency of solar energy capture by green plants can be as much as 3–4%, the more effective photosynthetic plants – like maize, sorghum and especially sugar cane – being the most productive.

The current 'energy crisis' that is reverberating throughout the world has focused attention on the finite nature of fossil-fuel reserves. Taken in association with the dramatic increase in industrialisation in many developing countries, this has generated growing economic and trade pressures for cheaper and reliable supplies of energy. The only alternative regenerable supply of feedstocks for the chemical industry will be from the products of photosynthesis, i.e. sugar, starch and lignocellulose.

Biomass can be considered as a renewable energy source, and can be converted into either direct energy or energy-carrier compounds by direct combustion, anaerobic digestion systems, destructive distillation, gasification, chemical hydrolysis and biochemical hydrolysis.

6.2 Sources of biomass

There are three main directions that can be followed to achieve biomass supplies (Fig. 6.1):

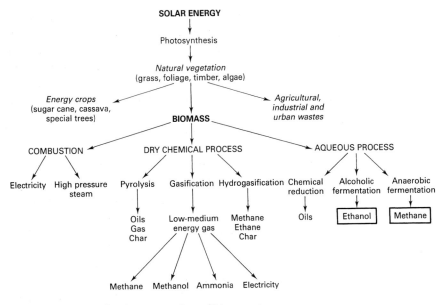

Fig. 6.1 Options for the conversion of biomass to energy.

(1) cultivation of so-called 'energy crops'
(2) harvesting of natural vegetation
(3) utilisation of agricultural and other organic wastes.

Many woody crops such as alder, willow and birch, which can be readily coppiced, can be grown to offer direct fuel sources to be used in power stations. Some success has already been achieved in Scandinavia. In other parts of Europe with considerable redundant farmland resulting from reductions in cereal cultivation, this land could be used for the cultivation of woody perennials or coppiced trees for fuel-energy production.

The conversion of biomass to usable fuels can be accomplished by biological or chemical means or by a combination of both. The two main end products are methane or ethanol, although other products may arise depending on initial biomass and the processes utilised, e.g. solid fuels, hydrogen, low-energy gases, methanol and longer-chain hydrocarbons.

The concept of cultivating plant biomass specifically for energy supply is based on the fact that much higher yields of fixed carbon are attainable from well-planned plantation methods than from harvesting natural vegetation or collecting agricultural or industrial wastes. Programmes of this type are now being extensively planned and practised in many countries throughout the world. Sugar cane and cassava are the two principal crops that are being developed (primarily for ethanol production) in Brazil, Australia and South Africa, whereas more lignocellulosic-based programmes are being developed in Sweden and America. In the latter case, plans are being made to grow forests for conversion into liquid fuels. Cost analysis of all of these processes offers considerable encouragement, in particular with sugar cane conversion.

Energy-crop plantations will undoubtedly supply meaningful amounts of energy in the near future. The problem of water deficiency is very real, however, and rainfall is most often the limiting factor operating in otherwise ideal conditions of solar radiation intensity, annual hours of sunshine, mild winters and an abundance of good-quality land. In certain areas of the world it is possible that such plantations will rapidly become a reality, but for most countries development will centre on the use of organic wastes – namely, agricultural, municipal and industrial. Conversion to biofuels could well serve as a substitute for petroleum energy and as a chemical feedstock.

The technical processing of the biomass depends on many factors, including moisture level and chemical complexity. With materials having a high water content, aqueous processing is normal to avoid the need for substrate drying. Alcoholic fermentation to ethanol and anaerobic digestion to methane, as well as chemical reduction to oily hydrocarbons, are all possible. Low moisture level materials such as wood, straw and bagasse can be: burnt to give heat or to raise steam for electricity generation; subjected to thermochemical processes such as gasification and pyrolysis to produce energy-rich compounds like gaseous oil, char and, eventually, methanol and ammonia; or treated by alkaline or biological hydrolysis to produce chemical feedstocks for use in further biological energy conversions.

While oil reserves rapidly decrease, and modern industry has not yet achieved any real capacity to change to alternative fuel, what realistic hopes can be placed on obtaining alternative fuels from biomass? Some of the leading methodologies will be examined.

6.3   Ethanol from biomass

The production of alcohol by fermentation of sugars and starch is an ancient art and is often considered to be one of the first microbial processes used by man.

$$C_6H_{12}O_2 \rightarrow 2CH_3CH_2OH + 2CO_2$$

Production of industrial alcohol by fermentation draws heavily upon the accumulated knowledge of the brewer and the distiller (Chapter 11). At present, industrial alcohol production is largely synthetic, i.e. non-microbial, deriving from petrochemical processes. Petrochemical ethanol is made by the hydration of ethylene, and the decline of microbial production of alcohol dates from the large-scale production of ethylene from the 1940s. Within 20 years of development of large-scale petroleum cracking, industrial production of fermentation alcohol fell below potable alcohol production in most industrialised nations. Thus, in technologically more advanced countries, ethanol is produced by chemical means. In many developing countries where cheap raw materials are available, ethanol is still produced for industrial purposes using traditional fermentation techniques.

While the benefits of ethanol as a fuel are considerable, i.e. it is energy efficient, does not produce toxic carbon monoxide during combustion and is, therefore, much less polluting than conventional fuels, it is still cheaper to produce ethanol from oil chemically than by fermentation processes at current oil prices. In this way, ethanol usage, as with other alternative fuels, is economically hindered in industrialised countries until oil prices once again take on an upward rise in price. It is inevitable that it will happen, but exactly when is hard to predict.

A dramatic change in the economics of alcohol production resulted from the massive increases in the world prices of crude oil in the 1970s. Whereas oil prices have more than quadrupled since 1975, the price of suitable cheap carbohydrates has risen far less on average.

Oil-importing nations are anxious to reduce their import costs and many now subsidise home-produced alternatives. Since alcohol can be used as a partial or complete substitute for motor fuel and can also be converted readily into ethylene and related compounds, its production from indigenous and renewable resources still seems an attractive alternative strategy.

Historically, ethanol and, to a lesser extent, methanol were used extensively as motor fuels in Europe prior to World War II and, indeed, Henry Ford's T model car was designed to run on alcohol, petrol or any mixture in between.

Nowhere has this been more actively pursued than in Brazil. Vast biotechnological processes operate throughout the country, converting sugar cane and cassava into ethanol by yeast fermentation. A production output of approximately 4×10^6 m^3 ethanol in the early 1980s has now been well surpassed. Brazil's ethanol programme is shown in Fig. 6.2. Brazil's undoubted success in pioneering this production of 'green petrol' has created worldwide interest, particularly amongst poorer developing nations with the climate and land to

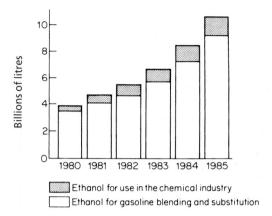

Fig. 6.2   The proposed ethanol programme for Brazil

grow their own fuel crops but with limited currency to buy oil. Even developed nations, such as Australia, the USA, Sweden and France, are embarking on biological alcohol production processes that utilise either large agricultural surpluses or forestry wastes.

Three billion litres of fuel alcohol were fermented in the USA from corn in 1987 and one-third of all American gasoline is 10% waste-derived ethanol or gasohol. Brazilian officials now estimate that the country's entire petrol needs could be met from planting 0.3% of the country's vast area with alcohol-producing crops. Over 500 fermentation and distillation plants have been built throughout the country, processing the crops produced throughout the year. An additional bonus to the energy generation is the creation of over 700 000 new direct jobs and 300 000 indirect jobs in the rural areas of Brazil.

However, the current economic scenario for Brazil's gasohol programme is being severely influenced by the current slump in world oil prices. By 1985, ethanol production had increased to 11 900 million litres, and by 1988, 88% of new cars were powered by ethanol engines. With the current world oil prices, production of ethanol has remained relatively static at about 11 000–12 000 million litres per year, and the government has ceased new financial investment. It is now realistically estimated that the costs of producing ethanol from sugar cane are at least US$50 per barrel.

Nevertheless, there are many indirect advantages to Brazil in using ethanol instead of gasoline. While there are obvious reductions in their contributions to global warming, the addition of anhydrous ethanol to gasoline eliminates the

Table 6.1. Potential raw materials for ethanol-fuel production

Starch containing	Cellulosics	Sugar containing	Other
Cereal grains	Wood	Sucrose and invert sweet sorghum	Jerusalem artichoke
Corn	Sawdust	Molasses	
Grain sorghum	Waste paper	Sugar beet	Raisins
Wheat	Forest residue	Fodder beet	Bananas
Barley	Agricultural residues	Sugar cane	
Milling products	Municipal solid wastes	Lactose	
		Whey	
Wheat flour	Intensive livestock		
Wheat mill feeds	Production wastes	Glucose	
Corn hominy feed		Sulphite wastes	
Starchy roots			
Mandioca			
Potatoes			

need for tetra-ethyl lead to raise the octane rating. Studies have further shown that ethanol-powered engines produce 57% less carbon monoxide, 64% less hydrocarbons and 13% less nitric oxides than gasoline-powered vehicles. Thus, while international oil prices continue to be low, the main justification for the continuation of bioethanol programmes must be environmental.

The world price of alcohol is still about twice that of oil, and fuel consumption is also up to 20% heavier with alcohol. However, these economic considerations are constantly changing in favour of alcohol production, with future anticipated increasing oil prices and new design concepts for alcohol-based engines. Furthermore, on a global aspect, green petrol production will help to take some of the pressure off oil products for the rest of the world, reducing competitive tensions and perhaps even wars.

Ethanol for fuel programmes requires a considerable capital investment and will be in keeping with large-scale needs and not small on-farm systems (where methane products are more suitable).

To make available the necessary fermentable sugars (Table 6.1), most raw materials require some degree of pre-treatment, depending on their chemical composition. With sugar cane, this treatment is minimal and consists mainly of the usual milling operation, whereas cassava roots (containing 25–38% starch on a wet-weight basis) require the action of a suitable saccharifying agent – either acid hydrolysis or enzyme hydrolysis. Cellulosic raw materials

Table 6.2. The gross energy requirements of ethanol produced from different substrates by microbial fermentation

Physical inputs	Substrates				
	Sugar cane	Cassava	Timber[a]	Timber[b]	Straw
Substrate	7.27	19.19	12.67	20.00	4.37
Additional chemicals	0.60	0.89	4.74	6.37	4.74
Water	0.30	0.38	0.80	0.30	0.80
Electricity	7.00	10.47	175.70	7.84	166.74
Fuel oil	8.00	29.03	42.13	62.40	42.13
Capital inputs (buildings, etc.)	0.46	1.21	3.34	0.64	3.34
Total	24	61	239	98	222

All figures given in MJ/kg ethanol.
[a] Fermentable sugars formed via enzymic hydrolysis.
[b] Fermentable sugars formed via acid hydrolysis.

such as timber and straw require more extensive pre-treatment, and this is reflected in the increased energy inputs required (Table 6.2). A flow diagram for the production of ethanol from diverse substrates is shown in Fig. 6.3.

The Brazilian programme is almost exclusively based on batch fermentation systems. At present, the standards of these fermentations are modest and leave much room for improvement. Continuous methods of production offer many advantages but are really only studied and operated in developed nations with an interest in ethanol formation. Improvements in continuous fermentations have utilised many approaches, including retention of the yeast cells in the bioreactor by separation and recycling and by continuous evaporation of the fermentation broth.

So far, innovation in the Brazilian programme has been restricted to some marginal improvements in essentially traditional alcohol fermentation processes. However, biotechnology is having a considerable input with new developments and numerous research programmes in this field, e.g. production of more efficient microorganisms by genetic engineering (improved alcohol fermentation, resistance to high temperatures and high alcohol levels, speed of fermentation and higher yields), by improved immobilised enzyme reactor technology, and by process design improvements. Novel introductions such as fermentation under partial vacuum and recycling of the fermentative yeast cells have increased ethanol productivity to 10 or 12 times that of conventional batch fermentation processes, and such increases reduce capital

ETHANOL

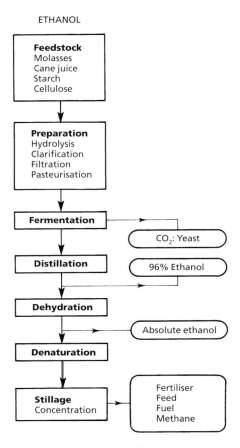

Fig. 6.3 Flow diagram for the production of ethanol.

costs and energy requirements for fermenter operation. Application of these biotechnological improvements to ethanol production will make these processes increasingly economically attractive as a substitute for fossil fuel.

The overall economics of fermenting ethanol from specific crop cultivation in developing countries will achieve support indirectly by the expansion of agriculture, by creating more employment, because oil prices will continue to outstrip agricultural feedstocks, and because new technologies will create further economic uses for the wastes generated in ethanol-fuel production.

Vast volumes of wastes or *stillage* result from the Brazilian and other alcohol programmes, and much research is in progress to seek worthwhile end products. Of particular significance will be:

(1) evaporation to feed or fertilisers;
(2) mineralisation to ash;
(3) anaerobic fermentation for methanol generation;
(4) conversion by microorganisms into SCP.

There can be no doubt that, eventually, oil price rises will make gasohol programmes advantageous in simple economic terms.

Recently there has been a growing interest in some parts of Europe in the use of modified rapeseed oil as a diesel substitute – *biodiesel*. Biodiesel is obtained from rapeseed as the result of a reaction between the oil and methanol in the presence of a catalyst such as sodium hydroxide at 50°C, producing an ester and glycerol.

Rapeseed oil + Methanol → Diester + Glycerol
(1 tonne)   (0.1 tonne)   (1 tonne) (0.1 tonne)

The glycerol is allowed to settle and the biodiesel purified and used as a fuel. The purified biodiesel has physical and chemical properties that are similar to those of diesel fuel and heating fuel oil. The use of biodiesel does not require any specific engine modifications.

What are the main advantages of biodiesel? Firstly, the energy yielded is considerably greater than that consumed during its production and will increase with improved (genetically engineered) cultivars of rapeseed. Secondly, it is non-toxic and more than 98% biodegradable, and its contribution to the greenhouse effect is three to five times less than that of diesel. Above all, it is renewable.

France, Italy and Germany have been the leading proponents of biodiesel – France for agricultural reasons, Italy for environmental reasons and Germany for both.

Many public urban transport systems in these countries burn biodiesel, thus enhancing their 'environmental' image. Italy has given preference to its use as a fuel for heating municipal buildings. In European countries a considerable amount of agricultural land must be 'set aside' or used for non-agricultural produce production. For this reason the growth of rapeseed as a fuel crop offers exciting commercial and environmental opportunities and almost all European countries have vested interests.

The wider application of diesel will depend on special fiscal measures. In the European Union, a draft directive is under consideration with the view to harmonising the various national fiscal requirements governing biofuels, with a suggested limit of excise rate of a maximum of 10% of the tax on fossil fuel. It has recently been suggested that ethanol from biomass could replace

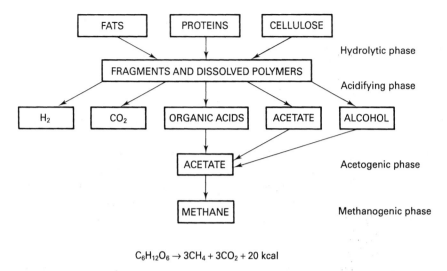

$$C_6H_{12}O_6 \rightarrow 3CH_4 + 3CO_2 + 20\ kcal$$

Fig. 6.4 The microbiology of methane generation.

the methanol of fossil origin used in the esterification reaction. In this way, bio-ethanol usage would be increased and the biodiesel would be derived from entirely renewable resources. The biodiesel market is real and will expand in the near future.

6.4   Methane from biomass

Methane gas can be used for the generation of mechanical, electrical and heat energy, and is now extensively used as a fuel source for domestic and industrial purposes through national gas pipelines or can be converted to methanol and used as fuel in internal combustion engines. Such natural gas sources were originally derived from biomass in ancient times.

Methane gas also exists in the atmosphere and is mainly derived from microbial action in natural wetlands, rice paddies and enteric fermentation in animals, contributing about 20%, 20% and 15% respectively to the total methane flux. Domestic cattle are the major contributors, producing about 75% of all animal emissions, whereas humans produce about 0.4%. After carbon dioxide, methane is considered to be the next most important greenhouse gas and is expected to contribute 18% of future warming.

The microbiology of methane production is complex (Fig. 6.4), involving mixtures of anaerobic microorganisms. In principle, anaerobic fermentation of complex organic mixtures is believed to proceed through three main bio-chemical phases, each of which requires specific microbiological parameters. The initial stage requires the solubilisation of complex molecules such as cellu-lose, fats and proteins, which make up most raw organic matter; the resultant soluble, low molecular weight products of this stage are then converted to organic acids. In the final phase of microbial activity, these acids (primarily acetic) are specifically decomposed by the methanogenic bacteria to methane and CO_2.

The most efficient and complex methane-producing system in nature is the rumen. This anaerobic system has never been fully reproduced outside the cow, and is known to be a complex interaction of large numbers of bacteria, protozoa and fungi. All intensively studied bioreactor programmes set up to create methanogenesis under controlled conditions have shown that consistently high gas outputs require substantial laboratory monitoring with highly accurate control of environmental variables such as temperature, pH, moisture level, agitation and raw material input and balance. To date, most practical applications of methanogenesis have been at a very low technological level.

There are several possible ways by which methane can be produced in a planned economy: from sewage, from agricultural and urban wastes, and in biogas reactors.

The anaerobic digestion of *sewage* is a long-practised technique and many municipal systems have devised methods of capturing the methane and har-nessing the energy for the needs of the sewage plant. The energy returns are modest and large-scale expansion does not seem probable (Chapter 9).

In recent years, methanogenesis of the abundantly available *agricultural and urban wastes* has appeared as an obvious and profitable way to generate energy. The energetic considerations of methane production from such wastes are complex and subject to many limitations. Using urban wastes it should be possible to convert 30–50% of the combustible energy to methane, while with the use of certain other vegetable materials or forages it may be possible to achieve 70% conversion. The overall economics of methane production must recognise the valuable by-products generated by the process, namely the effluent and residue rich in ammonia, phosphates and microbial cells, which may be used as fertiliser, soil conditioner or even as animal feed. Furthermore, the process can convert malodorous and pathogenic wastes into innocuous and useful materials.

However, there are still many inherent problems that must be overcome before there can be any hope of achieving an energy balance. At present, the cost of collection of organic matter only for the purpose of methanogenesis is too expensive; the rate of methane production is inconsistent and low in most processes, and much research needs to be carried out on the balance of nutrients for process optimisation. However, the major problem is the presence of lignin in most agricultural and urban wastes. Lignins are not easily digested by anaerobic processes, and physical and chemical pre-treatment places a considerable energy and cost burden on the overall process.

When methane is produced by the fermentation of animal dung, the gaseous products are usually referred to as '*biogas*' and the installations as 'biogas plants' or 'bioreactors'. Biogas is a flammable mixture of 50–80% methane, 15–45% carbon dioxide, 5% water and some trace gases. Biogas is produced via biomethanation (Fig. 6.4) and is in fact a self-regulating symbiotic microbial process operating under anaerobic conditions, and functions best at temperatures of about 30°C. The organisms involved are all found naturally in ruminant manures. In such systems the animal dung is mixed with water and allowed to ferment in near-anaerobic conditions. Production of biogas by such methods goes back into antiquity and is of particular importance in India, China and Pakistan. The Gobar system of biogas production in the Far East ranges from small peasant systems to quite large plants that continuously produce large volumes of gas. In energy terms, the simple Gobar system is very near to being a net energy producer on a small scale. Small-scale plants of family, farm or village size are in operation throughout the world.

Under ideal conditions, 10 kg dry organic matter can produce 3 m^3 of biogas, which will provide 3 h cooking, 3 h lighting or 24 h refrigeration with suitable equipment. Biogas does, in fact, furnish a considerable part of the world's energy source; China is the largest user, with over 7 million biogas units providing the equivalent energy of 22 million tons of coal, and with current subsidies, a biogas plant in China is cheaper than a bicycle. Larger systems of this type do not achieve a net energy balance.

Biogas combustion has been used to heat steam to drive electricity turbines, and in California, USA, one plant provides electricity to 20 000 homes by way of cow-manure biomethanation.

There has also been some consideration of growing crops on a large scale to provide a 'methane economy'. High-yielding crops (in terms of million joules/hectare/enthalpy, cultivated on massive land or water areas have been proposed. It has been suggested that 65% of the current gas consumption in the USA could be provided by an energy plantation of area 260 000 km^2 using water hyacinth of energy content 3.8 MJ/kg dry material. Marine algae have also come under special scrutiny.

Methane generated from organic materials by anaerobic fermentation offers a valuable source of energy that could be directly put to many uses.

Table 6.3. Economic arguments against large-scale methane production by microbial processes

---

(1) An abundance of methane occurs in nature, particularly in natural gas fields and oil field overlays.
(2) Methane production by gasification of coal is commercially more attractive.
(3) Microbial production of methane is more expensive than that of natural gas.
(4) On account of the costs of storage, transportation and distribution of gaseous fuels, large-scale production is not yet economically worthwhile.
(5) Methane cannot be used in cars and is difficult and expensive to convert to a liquid state.

Furthermore, the associated by-products may be useful forms of fertilisers for agriculture. Yet, before the full realisation of these systems can be achieved, very considerable biotechnological studies must be undertaken. The biological aspects revolve around complex mixed cultures and it is doubtful that the thermodynamic efficiency of the fermentation can be improved. Thus, emphasis must be given to improving process design and to technological improvements of the control systems. New and cheap construction materials for digesters (bioreactors) and gas storage vessels will be required. In time, there will be available a complete range of anaerobic technologies to deal with most kinds of biodegradable materials. Although methane will be the principal end product, fuels such as propanol and butanol, as well as fertilisers, will undoubtedly add to the cost-effectiveness of the overall process.

Methane as an energy source may well have economic value at local small-scale production levels, but there is considerable doubt about the future of large-scale commercial processes for methane production. Some of the more obvious considerations are shown in Table 6.3.

However, anaerobic digestion of municipal, industrial and agricultural wastes can have positive environmental value, since it can combine waste removal and stabilisation with net fuel (biogas) formation. The solid or liquid residues can further be used as fertiliser, soil conditioner or animal feed.

Biogas production will continue to have high priority in alternative energy research.

6.5 Hydrogen

Consideration has been given to the use of hydrogen as a fuel or in fuel cells for the production of electricity. Hydrogen production can occur by way of

Table 6.4. A typical oil well production scenario

Oil source	Original oil-in-place (%)
Produced	24.0
Reserves	8.8
Tertiary oil target	13.6
Future technically developed targets	13.6
Unrecoverable	40

photosynthetic bacteria, by biophotolysis of water and by fermentation. In the first two systems, encouraging production of hydrogen has been achieved, but much research is needed to assess the significance of these methods at an applied level. It has been estimated that at least 20–30 years of research is needed before any type of functional system is obtained.

Although it is possible to generate hydrogen from glucose by bacterial action, the production rate is too small to make microbial genesis of hydrogen economic.

The efficiency of hydrogen production by anaerobic fermentation is much less than that of methane production by the same method. Since methane also has a higher energy content, it would appear that methane production by microbial processes has a much higher practical potential than hydrogen. However, further research may well alter these considerations.

Although biomass may ultimately only supply a relatively small amount of the world's energy requirements (the estimate for the USA is approximately 5%), it will nevertheless be of immense overall value. In parts of the world such as Brazil, and countries of similar climatic conditions, biomass will surely attain wider exploitation and utilisation. The technical and agronomic problems are still considerable but biotechnological research is making valuable inroads to further understanding.

Although biomass may still have many disadvantages when compared with oil and coal, the very fact that it is renewable, and they are not, must be the spur to further research. In time, biomass will become much more easily and economically used as a source of energy.

6.6   Postscript: microbial recovery of petroleum

When an oil field is opened up, spontaneous and/or pumping will produce only about one-third of the total petroleum present. Secondary recovery techniques such as gas pressurising, water flooding, miscible flooding and thermal methods can further increase output. Tertiary oil recovery methods involving the use of solvents, surfactants and polymers that are able to dislodge oil from geological formations can further increase or prolong the production life of a well (Table 6.4). Microbially enhanced oil recovery processes involve the use of polymers such as xanthan gum, produced by large-scale fermentation of specific bacteria. Such gums have excellent viscosity and flow characteristics and can pass through small-pore spaces, releasing more trapped oil. Application is usually associated with water-flooding operations. A further possible approach is the use of microorganisms *in situ* for dislodging oil by way of surfactant production, gas formation or even altering the viscosity of the oil by partial microbial degradation. At present, the difficulties outweigh the disadvantages. Biosurfactants may also have a role in releasing oil from tar sands.

7

Single cell protein (SCP)

7.1 The need for protein

A major challenge to creating a sustainable future for the world's populations will be to secure adequate food supplies for the majority. The number of humans in the world now approximates six billion, and increasing, and could well be over nine billion within the next 25 years (Fig. 7.1). Fortunately, recent statistics suggest that world population growth rate is slowing but, even so, overall numbers are increasing. Patterns of births worldwide indicate that over 90% are occurring in the southern hemisphere, where already 80% of the world's population live, yet they only use 20% of the world's resources.

It is also estimated that, by 2030, urban populations will be at least twice that of rural populations. The growth of urbanisation, together with ensuing environmental degradation, causes serious losses in the availability of productive agricultural land. In many parts of the world, such as Africa, soil fertility is declining and is further exacerbated by increasing water scarcity in the southern hemisphere. Furthermore, worldwide climate changes and increasing civil strifes continue to make accurate predictions of future food supplies unpredictable.

It is becoming increasingly documented that conventional agriculture will struggle to supply sufficient food, in particular protein, to satisfy a growing world population.

However, productivity is increasing throughout the world in all branches of agriculture. Biotechnological innovations will accelerate this trend (Chapter 10). Food surpluses are occurring in many places, particularly in North America and western Europe, where there are near static populations.

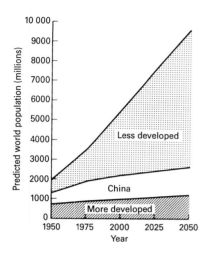

Fig. 7.1 Population totals.

Furthermore, some countries that had been net importers of major foods, such as India and Indonesia, are now self-sufficient. World supply of grain per head has outpaced population growth. However, there are still major imbalances in the availability of cereals; these are further disturbed by changes in global weather patterns (in particular rainfall) and by national and international warfare with ensuing disruption of agriculture and food distribution.

The extent of the protein problem varies from country to country and must be considered within the framework of each national economy. The shift from grain to meat diets in developed and developing countries is of dramatic proportions and is leading to a much higher per capita grain consumption, since it takes 3–10 kilograms of grain to produce 1 kilogram of meat by animal rearing and fattening programmes.

The search for sources of protein is relentlessly pursued. New agricultural practices are widespread: high-protein cereals have been developed; the cultivation of soya beans and groundnuts is ever-expanding; protein may be extracted from liquid wastes by ultrafiltration; and now the use of microbes as protein producers has gained wide experimental and commercial success. This field of study has become known as *single cell protein* production or 'SCP', referring to the fact that most of the microorganisms used as producers grow as single or filamentous individuals rather than as complex multicellular organisms like plants or animals.

Eating microbes may seem strange, but people have long recognised the nutritional value of some large microorganisms, such as mushrooms. However, even here, scepticism and prejudice have influenced people's attitudes, and while in some countries mushrooms are widely consumed, in others they are avoided and neglected. Although massive mushroom production processes are now commercially successful throughout the world, this chapter is largely concerned with the growth of more simple microorganisms, namely bacteria, yeast, filamentous fungi and algae, which lend themselves to biotechnological processing. Whereas mushroom growing, because of its antiquity, can be considered as a conventional type of food production, the use of other microbes is less appreciated and presents many problems, not all of which are technological in nature.

During the last two decades there has been a growing interest in using microbes for food production, in particular for feeding domesticated food-producing animals such as poultry. It has been argued that the use of SCP derived from low-value waste materials for animal feed would improve human nutrition, by taking protein-rich vegetable foods out of the human/animal competition and making them more freely available for human consumption in the producer countries, which are often developing countries. Many major companies throughout the world have long been actively involved in these SCP processes, and many worthwhile products are commercially available.

Protein quality and quantity are the goals of SCP production. However, the microbes also contain carbohydrates, fats, vitamins and minerals, and produce them from (in general) otherwise inedible or low-quality waste materials.

SCP may be used as a protein supplement for humans and animals. With humans it has been considered as a protein supplement, as a food additive to improve flavour and fat binding, and more recently as a replacement for animal protein in the diet. Because humans have a limited capacity to degrade nucleic acids, additional processing is required before SCP can be used in human foods. Microorganisms have high DNA/RNA contents, and human metabolism of nucleic acids yields excessive amounts of uric acid, causing kidney stones and gout! In animal feeding it can serve as a replacement for such traditional protein supplements as fishmeal and soymeal. The high protein levels, bland odour and taste of SCP, together with ease of storage, confer considerable potential to SCP in food and food outlets. Its high protein content makes its use attractive in aquaculture, e.g. farming shrimps, prawns, trout and salmon.

Microorganisms produce protein much more efficiently than any farm animal (Table 7.1). The protein-producing capacities of a 250-kg cow and 250 g of microorganisms are often compared. Whereas the cow will put on 200 g of protein per day, the microbes, in theory, could produce 25 tonnes in the same time under ideal growing conditions. However, the cow also has the unique ability to convert grass into protein-rich milk. After decades of research, no rival method for that conversion process has been developed.

Table 7.1. The time required to double the mass of various organisms

Organism	Time required to double mass
Bacteria and yeasts	20–120 minutes
Moulds and algae	2–6 hours
Grass and some plants	1–2 weeks
Chickens	2–4 weeks
Pigs	4–6 weeks
Cattle (young)	1–2 months
Humans (young)	3–6 months

Table 7.2. The advantages of using microbes for SCP production

Microorganisms can grow at remarkably rapid rates under optimum conditions; some microbes can double their mass every 0.5–1 hour.

Microorganisms are more easily modified genetically than plants and animals; they are more amenable to large-scale screening programmes to select for higher growth rate, improved acid content, etc., and can be more easily subjected to gene transfer technology.

Microorganisms have relatively high protein content and the nutritional value of the protein is good.

Microorganisms can be grown in vast numbers in relatively small continuous-fermentation processes, using relatively small land area, and are also independent of climate.

Microorganisms can grow on a wide range of raw materials, in particular low-value wastes, and some can also use plant-derived cellulose.

The cow has recently been described as 'a live, self-reproducing and edible bioreactor'.

The advantages of using microbes for SCP production are outlined in Table 7.2.

7.2 Acceptability and toxicology of SCP

A unique aspect of the SCP field is the extent to which it has been influenced by factors other than purely technological or economic ones. Geographic, political, sociological and psychological influences have shaped the course of development to a very marked degree. In particular, a tremendous amount of attention has been given to the problems of safety, nutritional value and acceptability of the product.

The nature of the raw materials used in SCP processes represents the main safety hazard, for example the possibility of carcinogenic hydrocarbons in the gas oil or n-paraffins, of heavy metals or other contaminants in the mineral salts, of solvent residues after extraction, and of toxin production (mycotoxins) by certain fungi. The process organism must be non-pathogenic and non-toxigenic and the products of the organism's metabolism must be innocuous. Rigorous sanitation and quality control procedures must be maintained throughout the process to avoid spoilage or contamination by pathogenic or toxigenic microorganisms.

Toxicological testing of the final product must include short-term acute toxicity testing with several different laboratory animal species, followed by extensive and detailed long-term studies – 2 years or more – in both rodent and non-rodent species. All in all, it represents a major scientific and financial investment, but after the thalidomide disaster, when a drug taken to suppress the nausea of 'morning sickness' caused foetal limb abnormalities, it is better to err on the side of caution.

The acceptability of SCP when presented as a human food depends not only on its safety and nutritional value, but also on other factors. In addition to the general reluctance of people to consume material derived from microbes, the eating of food has many subtle psychological, sociological and religious implications. In various cultures there are many specific associations related to eating and status and symbolic values are attributed to different kinds of food. More obvious factors influencing acceptability must be considered, such as odour, colour, taste and texture. Thus, if SCP is to be used directly as human food, the skills of the food technologist will be greatly challenged. Most realistic considerations would place SCP for human food at a relatively low priority. Demand will mainly be as a food source for various types of domesticated animals, poultry and fish. However, some industrial processes will be primarily directed to human consumption, e.g. Rank-Hovis-McDougall/ICI fungal protein ('Quorn'), which is gaining an increasing market place as a vegetable protein with meat-like texture and appearance.

What about the political and sociological influences on the production of SCP? These problems have mainly centred around the use of oil-derived materials as substrate for SCP. Such 'petro-proteins' have been suspected of being contaminated with carcinogens; consequently, massive SCP programmes in Japan, Italy and Britain were abandoned and efforts re-directed to the study of alcohol-methanol-based SCP and SCP from organic wastes.

The critical parameters of SCP processes are strongly interdependent. The choice of substrate will reflect local political and economic factors and the availability of alternative outlets. The choice of organism will partly determine the process technology and the nature of the product. Acceptability of product will depend in part on the substrate. On account of the large volumes that will be involved in SCP processes, continuous-culture techniques will be widely selected for economic reasons. Most large concerns actively involved in SCP production have based their processes on such techniques.

7.3   SCP derived from high-energy sources

Materials with a high commercial value as energy sources or derivatives of such chemicals, e.g. gas-oil, methanol, ethanol, methane and *n*-alkanes, have found wide commercial interest. The microbes involved are mostly bacteria and yeasts and several processes are now in operation. As would be expected, most oil companies have been, or are still, involved in this field. The wisdom of using such high-energy potential compounds for food production has been questioned by many scientists.

Methane as an SCP source has been extensively researched but is now considered to present too many technical difficulties to warrant exploitation.

In contrast, methanol offers great economic SCP interest. A large-scale (75 000 litre) fermentation plant for producing the methanol-utilising bacterium *Methylophilus methylotrophus* was constructed by ICI, UK. Hoechst (West Germany) and Mitsubishi (Japan) worked on a similar process, using yeast strains instead of bacteria. The ICI SCP protein (named 'Pruteen') was used exclusively for animal feeding. Methanol as a carbon source for SCP has many inherent advantages over *n*-paraffins, methane gas and even carbohydrates: composition is independent of seasonal fluctuations; there are no possible sources of toxicity in methanol; methanol dissolves easily in the aqueous phase in all concentrations; and no residue of carbon source remains in the harvested biomass. Several other important technical aspects are also very relevant.

The ICI Pruteen plant was the only process of its kind in the western world but could not operate economically at present methanol prices and has ceased production. Methanol represents approximately 50% of the cost of the product. In the USA, the cost of SCP derived from methanol is two to five times the cost of fishmeal. In the Middle East, the low cost of methanol and higher costs of fishmeal, coupled with a need to produce more animal products, could make SCP an attractive proposition. In the former Soviet-bloc countries, many methanol plants are operated. In part this is due to chronic shortages of animal feeds, excess production of methanol, lack of foreign currency to buy alternatives such as soyabean meal and, above all, a disregard for economic planning. However, political and economical changes in Russia have led to many closures of SCP production plants. Currently soyameal retails at about $300 per tonne and fishmeal at $400–450 on the basis of protein content and quality.

The vast range of studies carried out in the 1960s to 1970s on the potential use of methanol and related compounds as substrates for SCP processes certainly pushed bioreactor technology to its limits for cheap bulk-product formation. The aerobic process for Pruteen production was the world's largest continuous bioprocess system. The stringent economies required in these processes led to extensive use of airlift bioreactor design. Furthermore, the massive volume and expense in harvesting and preparing the final product forced many economies of scale and of downstream processing. At its peak in Russia, there were several SCP plants on stream or being planned with production capacity of 300 000–600 000 tonnes per annum.

Ethanol is a particularly suitable source if the SCP is intended for human consumption. In the foreseeable future the comparative status of ethanol SCP will depend on local factors: over-capacity in ethylene crackers, agricultural carbohydrate surpluses, and political decisions about regional economic independence and foreign trade balances.

The use of *n*-alkanes as a substrate for SCP has been extensively studied in many countries and represents a very complex biotechnological process. However, most of these processes have now ceased operation because of suspected health hazards resulting from the presence of carcinogens in the SCP. More recently, however, the massive technology developed in this field in Japan and other eastern countries has been turned over to the study of alcohol-based SCP and SCP from organic wastes.

7.4   SCP from wastes

The materials that make up wastes should normally be recycled back into the ecosystem, e.g. straw, bagasse, citric acid, olive and date wastes, whey, molasses, animal manures and sewage. The amount of these wastes can be locally very high and may contribute to a significant level of pollution in water courses. Thus, the utilisation of such materials in SCP processes serves two functions – reduction in pollution and creation of edible protein. Of particular interest has been the extensive programmes to convert cattle and pig wastes to feed

Table 7.3. Advantages of using widely available organic wastes for SCP production

It reduces environmental pollution.
Most organic wastes are available at low cost in most countries, thus ensuring independence in supply.
The wastes are upgraded in energy and protein level.
It guards against a protein shortage in a community that may be largely dependent on imports.
It allows for technological innovation, which can often be transferred to developing countries.
Many of the wastes, such as cellulose and whey, already form accepted parts of animal diets and will avoid the acceptability problems of other unusual wastes, e.g. human wastes and fossil fuels.

protein. However, these studies have been largely unsuccessful due to technical and sanitary difficulties.

An attractive feature of carbohydrate waste as a raw material is that, if its low cost can be coupled with suitable low process costs, an economic SCP product may be obtained from relatively small operative units. The worldwide trend towards stricter effluent control measures, and parallel increases in effluent disposal charges, lead to the concept of waste as a negative-cost raw material. However, the waste may not be suitable for SCP or its composition, or dilution may be so dispersed that transport to a production centre may be prohibitive.

Each waste material must be assessed for its suitability for conversion to SCP. In particular, the level of available technology is important. When a waste is available in large quantities, and preferably over a prolonged time, then a suitable method of utilisation can be planned (Table 7.3).

SCP processes utilising waste substrates have been carried out on a commercial scale using various yeast organisms in sophisticated bioreactor systems. Substrates used and producer organisms include molasses (*Saccharomyces cerevisiae*) and cheese whey (*Kluyveromyces fragilis*), while the Symba process developed in Sweden utilises starchy wastes by combining two yeasts – *Endomycopsis fibuligira* and *Candida utilis*.

The feed value of the yeast produced by the Symba process has been evaluated in vast feeding experiments on different types of animals, including pigs, chickens and calves. The animals grew well and no adverse effects were recorded. The Symba process can be conveniently separated into three phases:

Phase 1. Waste water (from, for example, a potato processing plant) containing starch is fed through a heat exchanger and sterilised by steam injection.

Phase 2. Sterilised starch solution is fed through two bioreactors together with the starch-hydrolysing yeast *Endomycopsis fibuligira*. The hydrolysed starch then passes into a large bioreactor with *Candida utilis* as the growing organism.

Phase 3. The harvest stream from the *Candida* bioreactor is passed through vibro-screening and hydrocycloning equipment, then centrifuged. The samples collected can be spray dried and the dried material sifted and bagged or stored in bulk.

Pekilo was a fungal protein product that was produced by fermentation of carbohydrates derived from spent sulphite liquor, molasses, whey, waste fruits, and wood or agricultural hydrolysates. It had a good amino acid composition and was rich in vitamins. Extensive animal-feeding test programmes showed that Pekilo protein was a good protein source in the diet of pigs, calves, broilers, chickens and laying hens. Pekilo protein was produced by a continuous fermentation process. The organism, *Paecilomyces variotii*, a filamentous fungus, gave a good fibrous structure to the final product. However, the process does not appear to be in commercial operation at the present time.

In Britain, Rank-Hovis-McDougall, in conjunction with ICI (Marlow Foods), are now commercially marketing another fungal protein – mycoprotein or 'Quorn' – derived from the growth of a *Fusarium* fungus on simple carbohydrates. Unlike almost all other forms of SCP, mycoprotein is produced for human consumption.

The use of abundantly available waste starch and sugars as a source of raw material for an SCP process was considered in the early 1960s by the late Lord Rank (then Chairman, Rank-Hovis-McDougall group of companies) to be a feasible and worthwhile project to alleviate the anticipated world protein famine. Under the direction of the late Professor Gerald Solomons, a 'starch into protein' process was commenced, which ultimately was to become the only successful SCP process developed entirely with human consumption as the primary aim. Three criteria were considered essential for this new food: (1) it must be 'delicious to eat', (2) the final product, the substrate and all possible intermediates used in the process must be safe to eat, and (3) above all, the final food presented should be highly nutritious.

Because the final product would require to be textured, bacteria would be unsuitable and filamentous fungi became the obvious choice. While starch was the initial best available substrate, it was considered that for a good controlled fermentation it would be necessary to use a soluble carbohydrate produced by the hydrolysis of starch. The fungus finally chosen was a *Fusarium*, and this was followed by an extensive fermentation programme that led ultimately to a novel continuous process.

This process can only be economic if operated on a continuous basis, and is routinely utilised for periods of several weeks without significant interruption and without contamination. The productivity, yield, composition and morphology of the organism are maintained steadily by careful regulation of the operating conditions.

The final fermentation product is pale-buff in colour, bland to taste, highly nutritious and fibrous in composition. It is now texturised by food scientists into meat-like analogues and, with correct culinary ingredients, can give a remarkable similarity to meat and chicken dishes. The process involved an extensive and prolonged safety and nutritional assessment, and since it was the first of its kind, this was to be the 'trend setter'. Unrestricted clearance was given by the UK ministry in 1985.

The production process and the marketing of the mycoprotein has been highly successful and production sites should become worldwide in the very near future. At the present time this is the only liquid fermentation-derived microbial SCP process for human food production that is economically operated in the world.

The research and approval of the Rank-Hovis-McDougall *Fusarium* SCP mycoprotein is estimated to have cost over \$40 million and the duration of the project was over a 20-year period. The original process was batch but was then developed into a continuous culture. The historical development of the process is shown in Fig. 7.2 and highlights not only the production of the fungal biomass but the equally important human and animal trials, the necessary food science required in formulation and presentation, and the development of market strategies.

The merger between Rank-Hovis-McDougall and ICI has ensured that the advanced technology developed by ICI for the now uneconomical Pruteen process is used to produce large quantities of the fungal protein. The product has had an excellent response from the public. A typical composition of mycoprotein compared with beef is shown in Table 7.4.

There can be little doubt that cellulose from agriculture and forestry sources and from wastes must constitute the future major feedstock for many biotechnological processes, including SCP. Cellulose, in its more natural association with lignin, is by far the most prevalent organic material available for biotechnological conversion. Throughout the world, research teams are studying ways

Table 7.4. Typical composition of mycoprotein in comparison with beef

Component	Mycoprotein	Raw lean beefsteak
Protein	47%	68%
Fat	14%	30%
Dietary fibre	25%	Trace
Carbohydrate	10%	0%
Ash	3%	2%
RNA	1%	Trace

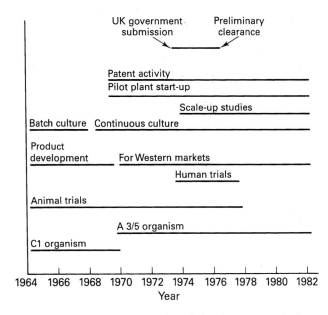

Fig. 7.2 Twenty-year research and development cycle for mycoprotein (courtesy of RHM Research Ltd).

of pre-treatment to disrupt or destroy the lignin barrier, and many physical and chemical methods have been examined (Table 7.5).

Next to cellulose, lignin is the earth's second most abundant natural biopolymer found in plants. Approximately 30% of most woody plants is composed of lignin, and its catabolism and utilisation as a renewable resource are of great commercial interest. The natural abundance of lignin ensures that its biodegradation constitutes a vital part of the biophasic carbon cycle. The

Table 7.5. Strategy for the utilisation of complex lignocellulose wastes for SCP production

Factor	Process
Substrate preparation	Pre-treatment of the substrate *Physical*: milling techniques *Chemical*: short acid, alkaline or solvent treatment *Microbial*: screening for rotting organisms
	Hydrolysis of substrate *Chemical*: complete saccharification, with acid or alkali *Enzymatic*: production of cellulases, hemi-cellulases, etc. *Microbial*: screening for good microbial enzyme producers
Selection and improvement of microorganisms	
Selection of fermentation systems	Scale-up, optimisation of equipment, process control, batch or continuous process, preservation of final product
Nutritional and toxicological aspects	Chemical composition, animal feeding tests, acceptability, toxicology
Economics	Cost analysis, comparative considerations with other materials, energy balances

elucidation of the lignin biodegradation process is essential to understanding the circumstances for the recycling of carbon on earth, for establishing the technology for bioconversion of plant residues and waste lignins to useful materials (including edible biomass), and for the protection of the enviornment from lignin-derived pollutants.

A limited number of fungi and bacteria have the necessary enzymatic activities for lignin degradation. The major group of fungi to degrade woody materials, and especially the lignin component of lignocellulosics, is the white-rot basidiomycetes. The fungus *Phanerochaete chrysosporium* is one of the most studied lignin degraders and is considered to have great potential for future biotechnological applications. Arising from these biochemical studies, scientists now have a better understanding of the structures and breakdown mechanisms for lignin biodegradation.

Table 7.6. World production of cultivated edible and medicinal mushrooms in different years

Species	1981 Metric tons	%	1990 Metric tons	%	1997 Metric tons	%
			Fresh wt $\times$ 10^3			
Agaricus bisporus/ bitorquis	900.0	71.6	1420.0	37.8	1955.9	31.8
Lentinula edodes	180.0	14.3	393.0	10.4	1564.4	25.4
Pleurotus spp.	35.0	2.8	900.0	23.9	875.6	14.2
Auricularia spp.	10.0	0.8	400.0	10.6	485.3	7.9
Volvariella volvacea	54.0	4.3	207.0	5.5	180.8	3.0
Flammulina velutipes	60.0	4.8	143.0	3.8	284.7	4.6
Tremella spp.	—	—	105.0	2.8	130.5	2.1
Hypisizygus spp.	—	—	22.6	0.6	74.2	1.2
Pholiota spp.	17.0	1.3	22.0	0.6	55.5	0.9
Grifola frondosa	—	—	7.0	0.2	33.1	0.5
Others	1.2	0.1	139.4	3.7	518.4	8.4
Total Increasing %	1357.2	100.0	3763.0	100.0	6158.4	100.0

From Chang (1999b).

Other basidiomycetes or mushroom-type fungi have long been shown to grow on lignocellulosic materials such as wood and straws and to produce edible mushrooms. The cultivation of edible mushrooms is one of the limited examples of a microbial culture in which the cultivated microorganism itself – i.e. the macroscopic, highly developed mushroom structure – is used directly as a human food. Mushroom cultivation also provides one of the few examples of successful commercial biotechnology processes based on lignocellulose as a substrate. A wide range of edible mushrooms are now cultivated through-out the world (Table 7.6) for human consumption. This solid-substrate fermentation (Chapter 4) is now one of the most challenging and technically demanding of all vegetable cultivations known to man. On a worldwide basis, mushroom growing is one of the fastest growing biotechnological industries (Fig. 7.3) and it is expected that it will expand even further with the production of enzymes and pharmaceutical compounds such as anti-cancer and anti-diabetic compounds.

The cultivation of the common white mushroom, *Agaricus bisporus*, has expanded worldwide and the USA continues to be the world's largest producer.

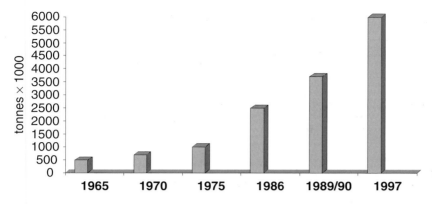

Fig. 7.3 Annual world production of cultivated edible mushrooms.

However, mushrooms traditionally grown in the Far East, such as *Lentinula edodes* (the Shiitake mushroom) and *Pleurotus* spp. (the oyster mushroom), are now expanding into other areas of the world, largely because of their unique flavours and textures and recognised medicinal qualities.

Mushroom production is, in principle, a fermentation process. In the case of *Agaricus*, the substrate for growth is fermented straw, while for *Lentinula* it is wood. For *Agaricus* cultivation the straw is composted with animal manures and other organic nitrogen compounds over a period of 1–2 weeks, and the final product is a unique substrate suitable for the rapid growth of the *Agaricus* inoculum. There is no standard pattern for compost formulation, being based only on the availability and price of the raw materials and supplements in the particular growing region. The nature of the substrate and its pre-treatment – more than all other aspects of growing – determine the method by which specific mushrooms are grown. When the mushroom mycelium has grown throughout the prepared compost (usually contained in large wooden boxes), the environmental conditions of temperature and humidity are altered, and subsequently the large mushroom structure rapidly forms in large numbers or 'flushes'. These are then harvested by hand cutting, and approximately 7–10 days later another crop will appear. Usually up to four crops are produced before the process is terminated. The cultivations of *Volvariella* and *Pleurotus* are again straw-based but have a much simpler procedure.

Lentinula edodes is the second most cultivated mushroom in the world and has been cultivated for over 1000 years. Currently, over 90% of its production occurs in Japan, but cultivation extends to China, Korea, Singapore, Taiwan, Sri Lanka and, more recently, into USA and Europe. The traditional method of cultivation has been to inoculate wooden logs (6′ × 0.5′) with spore inoculum

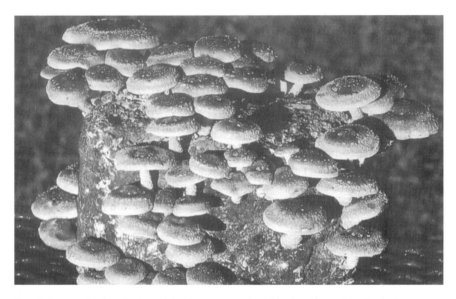

Fig. 7.4 *Lentinula edodes* cultivation on sawdust blocks. Since the plastic bags were removed at a later stage of mycelial development, most of the mushrooms appeared on the top (courtesy of Dr Myra Chu-Chou).

or mycelial plugs, allow the logs to stand for up to 9 months to achieve colonisation by the fungus, and then, during subsequent early summer and autumn periods, the mushrooms will grow out and be harvested. This seasonal production is augmented by drying mushrooms to achieve all-year-round consumption. The fungus derives its total nutrition from the lignocellulose of the log.

More recently, a new method of cultivation has been developed in which deciduous sawdust is mixed with cereal supplements and compressed into large plastic bags – artificial log production. The bags are sterilised and then inoculated aseptically with the pure fungus culture and, after a period of vegetative growth, are induced to produce the mushroom (Fig. 7.4). This controlled form of cultivation is leading to a wider geographical range of commercial cultivation not only for *Lentinula* but also for many other cultivated mushroom species.

Undoubtedly, the great advantage of these mushroom fermentations is the possibility of converting industrial, urban and wood wastes into a product which is directly edible by humans. However, irrespective of public demand and relative nutritional values, the future outlook for these processes will largely be related to the economics of production methods.

Biotechnological innovation is only now seriously being involved in this field, but the rewards will be great. Biotechnology need not always be high technology. To developing nations, where highly expensive systems may be impractical from the point of view of cost and lack of skilled operators, many of the new biotechnological discoveries may well lead to improvements in traditional microbial processes.

Major examples of solid-substrate fermentation are the many types of Oriental food fermentations. In many of these processes, bland materials such as beans, bran, etc., are subjected to microbial activity, to hydrolysing starch and proteins, and to creating products with basically enhanced flavours. Examples are traditional foods such as miso, shoyu, tempeh and many more local fermentations. Although many of these microbial-based foods are produced on a small cottage scale, others are the basis of large industries demanding major biotechnological inputs. Such foods and flavours are slowly becoming recognised in the West and will surely become a more acceptable part of our daily food intake.

7.5   SCP from agricultural crops

The previous section described how microorganisms can be used to produce SCP from organic waste such as sugars, starch and cellulose. Why not grow certain plants specifically as substrates for SCP processes? The concept of plant-biomass production as a feedstock for biotechnological processes is important as much higher yields of fixed carbon are attainable using a well-planned, preconceived plantation method than by harvesting natural vegetation or collecting crops or process wastes. At present, such programmes are practised largely for ethanol production, and it is thought that cassava, sugar cane and tapioca palm represent the only crops upon which it is likely that a mainstream fermentation operation could be economically established. When lignocellulose can be economically utilised, most parts of the world will have a readily renewable feedstock available for countless processes.

7.6   SCP from algae

There has been some interest in the use of algae as SCP since they grow well in open ponds and need only CO_2 as a carbon source and sunlight as an energy source for photosynthesis. Algae such as *Chlorella* and *Senedesmus* have long been used as food in Japan while *Spirulina* is widely used in Africa and Mexico.

Spirulina maxima is commercially produced in Mexico as a by-product of a large solar evaporator used for production of soda lime. Up to 2 tonnes per day are produced and used as animal feed. *Chlorella* is used as a protein and vitamin supplement in some Japanese yoghurts, ice cream and breads. In some parts of the world, algae are used in ponds or lagoons to aid in the removal of organic pollution, and the resultant biomass is harvested, dried and the powder added to animal feed.

7.7   The economic implications of SCP

The economic feasibility of SCP, apart from mushroom production, will be dictated by possible uses in competition with comparable existing products. SCP is protein-rich and can be stored and shipped over long distances. Its principal use will be as animal fodder, partly replacing other protein-rich materials such as soyabean meal or fishmeal. Being biological in the true sense, even though carried out industrially, these processes do not imbalance natural ecosystems. No novel synthetic compounds are produced and the technology – being based on recycling – is pollution-free.

SCP processes are mostly capital- and energy-intensive, and most processes must be conducted under sterile conditions in expensive equipment that can be cleaned and sterilised. The final product must not be exposed to microbial contamination, particularly human pathogens. To achieve economies of scale, SCP processes should have an input of at least 50 000 tonnes per year unless operated as a waste-treatment facility in a food processing plant. Thus, a considerable volume of raw materials must be nearby to meet these production requirements. Water requirements for SCP production are considerable for both processing and cooling.

The worldwide, large-scale development of SCP processes has contributed greatly to the advancement of present-day biotechnology. Research and development into SCP processes has involved work in the fields of microbiology, biochemistry, genetics, chemical and process engineering, food technology, agriculture, animal nutrition, ecology, toxicology, medicine and veterinary science, and economics. In developing SCP processes, new technical solutions for other related technologies have been discovered, e.g. in waste-water treatment, alcohol production and other metabolites, enzyme technology and nutritional sciences.

There is little doubt that the main short-term impetus for SCP production will come from the increasing legislative requirement for the disposal of both solid and liquid wastes in a manner that would be compatible with the preservation of the environment. The competitiveness of SCP for animal feed will improve when charges for effluent treatment are allowed for. The main reason for uncertainty with regard to profitability is undoubtedly the price of reference proteins, e.g. soyabean meat and fishmeal.

The future of SCP will be heavily dependent on reducing production costs and improving quality. This may be achieved with lower feedstock costs, improved fermentation and downstream processing, and improvement in the producer organisms as a result of conventional applied genetics together with recombinant DNA technologies.

However, the main limitations to the use of most SCP products for human use are sociological rather than technical, and consequently, in most cases the major nutritional role of microbial biomass or SCP will be as animal feed supplements.

8

Biotechnology and medicine

8.1 Introduction

During the twentieth century there have been the greatest gains in health in most parts of the world owing to dramatic reductions in infant mortality, eradication of life-threatening diseases such as smallpox, and considerable improvements in life expectancy in developing and industrialised countries. In the past, life for most people was coarse, lacking in adequate nutrition, with poor housing and, above all, short in years. With the advent of improved sanitation and better living conditions, together with the availability of vaccinations and antibiotics, there has been, for many, a vast improvement in health status. However, health status still differs widely among nations and by geographic region. For instance, life expectancy is less than 50 years in some sub-Saharan African countries, but over 75 years in established industrialised countries. The wealthiest economies appear to be the healthiest. A crucial factor related to life expectancy is access to safe water! In much of the developing world, simply drinking water is a high-risk exposure.

Undoubtedly, the real gains in health over the last century can be attributed mainly to the impact of public health and disease prevention rather than to medical interventions. Public health can be primarily distinguished from clinical medicine by placing emphasis on the prevention of disease rather than the curing, and having a main focus on population and communities rather than on the individual patient. It is essential to continue to develop a public health approach that will protect populations and create prevention strategies for groups and not just for individuals. Biotechnology has, and continues to play, a major part in establishing programes for achieving clean drinking water and waste-treatment technology (Chapter 9).

Nowadays in industrialised societies, infectious diseases are no longer the main threat to life; rather, it is the chronic diseases (cancer, cardiovascular disease, Alzheimer's disease, etc.) that plague our increasingly ageing population. Much of the increased life span achieved in the last 50 years has not prolonged youth but extended dotage. The late John F. Kennedy said in the 1960s: 'It is not enough for a great nation to have added new years to life. Our objective must be to add new life to those years.' Addressing the new problems of an ageing population will be a major challenge to modern medicine and biotechnology.

Chronic diseases will most probably not have a single, identifiable genetic cause but, rather, will arise from a complex, cascading series of biological events interacting with environmental factors. As indicated by Golub, 'the era of biology of specificity may rapidly be drawing to a close and we are entering the era of the *biology of complexity!*'. Consequently, biotechnology will increasingly be directed at maintaining normal human functions and a high personal level of health.

The impact of pharmaceuticals on human health care is an area where biotechnological innovations are likely to have the earliest commercial realisation. The long-standing awareness within the health-related industries of biological and biochemical innovations has led to these industries being heavily involved in biotechnological research, particularly molecular biology. Furthermore, since health-related products are generally of high value, the financial return warrants extensive research investment. Indeed, the majority of 'new' biotechnology investment over the last 30 years has been in health care, and especially in the discovery of new drugs. However, the considerable time required to develop a modern pharmaceutical product must not be underestimated, and long periods of toxicological testing are necessary before the national regulatory bodies will grant approval for marketing. The cost of achieving this approval can be many millions of pounds, and the product must have a high sales potential to warrant this investment. Many potentially worthwhile products will not appear on the market because it is not in the financial interest of the producing companies to meet such vast costs of gaining approval (Figs. 8.1 and 8.2).

New medical treatments based on new biotechnology are appearing almost daily in the marketplace. These include: (a) therapeutic products (hormones, regulatory proteins, antibiotics), (b) pre-natal diagnosis of genetic diseases, (c) vaccines, (d) immunodiagnostic and DNA probes for disease identification,

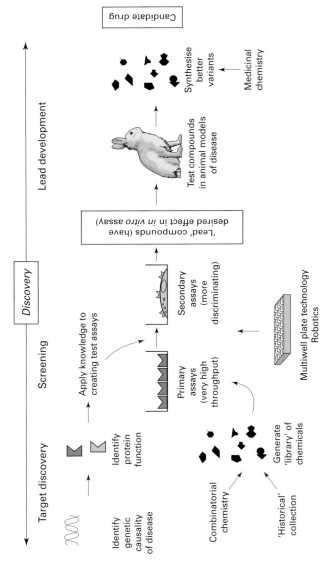

Fig. 8.1 Biotechnology drug discovery path. The process starts with genomics-driven discovery of a target gene and hence proteins, and with the generation of a diverse set of chemicals from combinational libraries or from collections of chemicals accumulated within a company. The chemicals are assayed for their ability to block (or sometimes enhance) the target protein's action (from Bains and Evans, 2001).

Candidate drug

Lead development

Discovery

Screening

Target discovery

Identify genetic causality of disease

Identify protein function

Apply knowledge to creating test assays

Primary assays (very high throughput)

Secondary assays (more discriminating)

'Lead' compounds (have desired effect in *in vitro* assay)

Test compounds in animal models of disease

Synthesise better variants

Medicinal chemistry

Multiwell plate technology Robotics

Combinatorial chemistry

'Historical' collection

Generate 'library' of chemicals

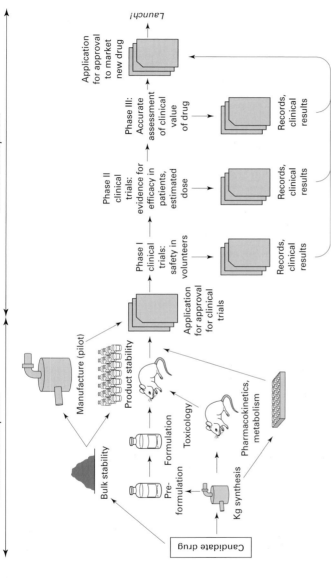

Fig. 8.2 Drug development path. The compound is formally tested for metabolism, toxicity, bioavailability and other pharmacological properties, traditionally in animals but increasingly in *in vitro* model assays. Successful compounds are then entered into an escalating series of clinical trials, producing systematic and extensive records which are used in the submission for permission to market the product as a drug (from Bains and Evans, 2001).

and (e) genetic therapy. This is the largest commercially developed area of new biotechnology, with massive present and future markets, and can only be selectively examined here.

8.2   Pharmaceuticals and biopharmaceuticals

The vast bulk of pharmaceutical drugs presently on sale are synthetic chemicals derived either directly by chemical synthesis or by chemically modifying molecules derived from biological sources. Biopharmaceuticals are considered as recombinant protein drugs, recombinant vaccines and monoclonal antibodies (for therapeutic roles). Biopharmaceuticals are becoming increasingly relevant in biological applications but are still only a small part of the pharmaceutical industry. However, there can be little doubt that the techniques of molecular biology/genetic engineering will become a dominating factor of drug discovery, design and development. Biotechnology will also accelerate screening, speed of bioassays and production of new drugs, and will also explain more accurately how drugs act in the human system. Biotechnology will almost certainly vastly reduce the huge costs presently incurred in the product development of new drugs (e.g. costs of discovery, development, scale-up, clinical trials and regulatory paperwork).

8.3   Antibiotics

The discovery in 1929 by Alexander Fleming that a fungus called *Penicillium notatum* could produce a compound that was selectively able to inactivate a wide range of bacteria, without unduly influencing the host, set in motion scientific studies that profoundly altered the relationship of humans to the controlling influence of bacterial diseases. Indeed, antibiotics changed forever the world in which we live. From these studies emerged the fungal antibiotics penicillin and cephalosporin, and the actinomycete antibiotics streptomycin, aureomycin, chloramphenicol, tetracyclines, and many others. Many bacterial diseases have largely been brought under control by the use of antibiotics. Pneumonia, tuberculosis, cholera and leprosy, to mention only a few, no longer dominate society and, at least in the developed parts of the world, have been relegated to minor diseases. Griseofulvin, an antibiotic active against fungi, has brought great relief to those infected with debilitating fungal skin diseases such as ringworm.

Table 8.1. Some economically important antibiotics

Antibiotic compound	Producer microorganism	Activity spectrum
Actinomycin D	*Streptomyces* sp.	Anti-tumour
Asparaginase	*Erwinia* sp.	Anti-leukaemia
Bacitracin	*Bacillus* sp.	Anti-bacterial
Bleomycin	*Streptomyces* sp.	Anti-cancer
Cephalosporin	*Acremonium* sp.	Anti-bacterial
Chloramphenicol	*Cephalosporium* sp.	Anti-bacterial
Daunorubicin	*Streptomyces* sp.	Anti-protozoal
Fumagillin	*Aspergillus* sp.	Amoebicidal
Griseofulvin	*Penicillium* sp.	Anti-fungal
Mitomycin C	*Streptomyces* sp.	Anti-tumour
Natamycin	*Streptomyces* sp.	Food preservative
Nisin	*Streptococcus* sp.	Food preservative
Penicillin G	*Penicillium* sp.	Anti-bacterial
Rifamycin	*Nocardia* sp.	Anti-tuberculosis
Streptomycin	*Streptomyces* sp.	Anti-bacterial

Antibiotics are antimicrobial compounds produced by living microorganisms, and are used therapeutically and sometimes prophylactically in the control of infectious diseases. Over 4000 antibiotics have been isolated, but only about 50 have achieved wide usage (Table 8.1). The other antibiotic compounds failed to achieve commercial importance for reasons such as toxicity to humans or animals, ineffectiveness or high production costs.

Antibiotics were extensively used in medicine from about 1945 with the arrival of penicillin. New antibiotics soon extended the range of antimicrobial control, and antibiotics are now widely used in human and veterinary medicine and (to a lesser extent) in animal farming, where some antibiotics have been shown to increase the weight of livestock and poultry. Antibiotics can also be used to a limited extent to control plant diseases and to act as insecticides.

Antibiotics that affect a wide range of microorganisms are termed '*broad spectrum*', e.g. chloramphenicol and the tetracyclines, which can control such unrelated organisms as *Rickettsia*, *Chlamydia* and *Mycoplasma* species. In contrast, streptomycin and penicillin are examples of '*narrow-spectrum*' antibiotics, being effective against only a few bacterial species. Most antibiotics have been derived from the actinomycetes and the mould fungi.

The production of antibiotics has undoubtedly been a highly profitable part of the pharmaceutical industries in the industrialised world. The world market for antibiotics is worth over $5 billion per year and is the most valuable segment of the total pharmaceutical market (about $200 billion). Due to biotechnology innovation, as world sales of antibiotics increase, their production costs decrease.

In 1992, the cephalosporins (products derived from cephalosporin C and penicillins G or V) were one of the largest business sectors in the global pharmaceutical market with sales at $8.3 billion. The present processes are highly efficient and have been achieved with little knowledge about the genetics of the producing organisms. This was, in part, due to the lack of an obvious sexual cycle, which limited cross-breeding experiments. However, new techniques such as protoplast fusion and gene transfer technologies are leading to the development of new strains with higher productivity and improved stability, and possible new products. These improvements have all resulted in continued decreases in overall costs of production. At present, all antibiotic fermentations involve centrally stirred tank reactors (Chapter 4) run under aerobic batch conditions. Modifications in production processes may well follow on from the novel fermenter designs that are gaining wider industrial acceptance.

It is regrettable to note that most studies on antibiotics have been concerned with diseases that are prevalent in the developed nations. Many diseases of developing countries, including many major tropical diseases, have received little attention from the major pharmaceutical industries. In part this may be due to the high level of technology, including specially trained personnel, that is normally associated with antibiotic research and development. More probably, the reason lies with the economics of developing new drugs for countries with limited financial resources. Let it be hoped that the advances in biotechnology may make it possible to follow a more enlightened pathway to develop the antibiotics necessary to combat the massive specific disease problems of the developing nations. Biotechnology may well make it possible to economically produce *orphan drugs* – drugs with specific needs but small profit return.

A disquieting observation has been the gradual evolution of drug resistance in many bacteria. As soon as antibiotics began to kill bacteria, bacteria began to evolve and change to disarm antibiotics. The possibility of this acquired resistance being transmitted to another species of bacterium is now real. For example, gonorrhoea (a venereal disease), which is resistant to treatment with penicillin, is now present in 19 countries. It is recognised that the resistance factors are located on plasmids within the bacterium and, because of this, can be more easily transmitted between organisms. The very core of gene transfer technology derives from this phenomenon. Antibiotic resistance in many well-known diseases is steadily increasing and must cause serious concern in our society. For example, TB, a former scourge of nations, had been nearly eradicated but is now increasingly being diagnosed in western countries! Hospitals are now infested with antibiotic-resistant bacteria such as methicillin-resistant *Staphylococcus aureus* (MRSA). Microorganisms can become resistant to antibiotics by way of several mechanisms. The exchange of genetic material between bacteria occurs frequently not just between like species but between diverse groups of bacteria. This consequently constitutes a global pool of resistant genes which are easily spread between different bacterial populations in man, animals and the environment.

The very large market for antibiotics in animal feeds and food preservation is now under considerable reappraisal. Without doubt, the addition of relatively small amounts of certain antibiotics (e.g. bacitracin, chlortetracycline, procaine, penicillin, etc.) in the feed of livestock and poultry led to the production of animals that were healthier, grew more rapidly and achieved marketable weight faster. However, there is now little doubt that the incorporation of medically important antibiotics into feed has led to increased spread of drug-resistant microorganisms, increased shedding of dangerous *Salmonella* bacteria in animal dung, and the transfer of antibiotic residues into human food.

As a consequence of the dangers of using antibiotics of human relevance in animal feed, there has been a massive effort to produce antibiotics specifically for animal feed incorporation, so replacing the medically used antibiotics. Thus, antibiotics of low therapeutic potency in humans or with an insufficient spectrum of activity are now more regularly used in animal nutrition.

While antibiotics continue to have a major role in the fight against microbial infections, antibiotics' resistance is now a disturbing concern for mankind. The cause of this lies mainly with the medical profession, with over-zealous prescribing and inappropriate applications of antibiotics for viral infection. There is, belatedly, more effort to educate doctors and the public on the inappropriate use of antibiotics. Sadly, there are still many countries that are not enlightened and continue to use antibiotics indiscriminately. Microbial populations do not respect national boundaries.

The clinical need for new antibiotics continues to grow and, while traditional screening protocols will continue, a more rational approach to new-antibiotic discovery could be the new availability of bacterial genome information. Functional genomics and proteomics as discussed earlier may bring new understanding to antibiotic resistance and, hopefully, new compounds will be designed to fight the microbes. Finally, biotechnology will continue to achieve new targets in manufacturing through fermentation yield improvements, recovery processes and final product purity.

8.4   Vaccines and monoclonal antibodies

According to the World Health Organization, each year more than 17 million people die from infectious diseases, preponderantly in the developing world. Human ingenuity has permitted mankind to protect itself against many infectious diseases through vaccination – a process which has been successful for more than a century. Central to the survival of humans and animals is the immune system. The immune system is composed of a series of organs, cells and molecules which are distributed throughout the body and which can function in concert, namely the innate (or non-specific) immune system and the acquired (or specific) immune system. The immune system provides a protective mechanism through which the body defends itself against invading organisms. The basic unit of immune function, the lymphocyte, is undoubtedly the most studied of all eukaryotic cells. Undoubtedly, immunology is at the centre of biomedical science, but yet remains a subject of great complexity.

During the last 20 years we have witnessed the unravelling of the bewildering processes of immune response in human and animal systems. When a foreign molecule (e.g. a microorganism) enters an animal system a remarkable chain of reactions is set in motion which, if successful, will result in the inactivation and exclusion of the invading microorganism. This molecular response can, in some cases, remain in the animal system for many years, giving complete or partial immunity against that type of microorganism. As discussed in Chapter 3, the foreign molecule is the *antigen*, which can elicit a counteracting response, the *antibody*, from the host system.

In general, antigens are proteins, or proteins combined with other substances such as sugars, though polysaccharides and other complex molecules may also act as antigens. In the disease process, antigens usually reside on the surface of the invading microorganism and trigger the body's defences against it. In this way antibodies are the essence of immunity against disease.

Antibodies are made by special cells throughout the body and it is now recognised that individual animal species, including humans, can produce unbelievable numbers of different antibodies. The antibody-producing cells recognise the shape of particular determinant groups of the antigen and produce specific antibodies in order to neutralise and eliminate the foreign substance. Thus, the human body has sufficient antibodies to combat not only the vast array of microbial invasions that can occur but also an unlimited range of synthetic chemicals. In short, the mammalian system can bind and inactivate almost any foreign molecule that gets in. However, should a particular antigen challenge not be dealt with adequately, then the invading microorganism can rapidly multiply and create imbalance, illness and perhaps death in the susceptible host.

The ability to stimulate the natural antibodies by vaccines has long been known. Vaccines are preparations of dead microorganisms (or fractions of them), or living attenuated or weakened microorganisms, that can be given to humans or animals to stimulate their immunity to infection. In this way they mimic infectious agents without the pathogenic consequences, and elicit in the body protective immune responses. When used on a large scale, vaccines have been a major force in the control of microbial diseases within communities. The major goals of vaccine research are to identify and characterise the individual antigens of infectious agents that elicit protective immune responses and to define the components in the immune response that induce protection.

Vaccines have been developed against many microbial diseases. However, the success and persistence of the antimicrobial effect vary widely between types of vaccines. Vaccines have eliminated smallpox from the world and polio from the northern hemisphere and have greatly reduced measles, rubella, tetanus, diphtheria and meningitis in many countries, saving countless millions of lives. Vaccines still remain the most cost-effective intervention available for preventing death and disease. However, there is a great disparity in their availability throughout the world. Reducing these differences between countries must be answered in the future. Vaccines must also be found for AIDS, malaria, tuberculosis, dysentery and other respiratory and diarrhoeal diseases. In excess of 30 million people will die of TB in the next decade, while the AIDS pandemic is causing devastation in many parts of the world, especially in the African continent.

Vaccine production is a high-cost, low-volume production system that encompasses many basic principles of biotechnology. Scale-up, in particular, is a constant problem when concerned with viral diseases that need to be produced from animal or human cell cultures. New advances in fermenter technology are rapidly revolutionising this work and should greatly increase vaccine production in the near future.

New methods of antibody production are now being considered. In current practice, antibodies are obtained from immunised animals, but this is usually a tedious and time-consuming operation. At the end of the various extraction and purification stages the antibodies are usually weakly specific, available only in small batches, and of variable activity. Attempts to culture antibody-secreting cells have been unsuccessful, since such cells neither survive for long enough nor produce enough antibodies in culture to become worthwhile sources of antibodies. Furthermore, such systems normally produce mixtures of different antibodies (polyclonal antibodies).

Table 8.2. Monoclonal antibody markets

(1) Cancer diagnosis and therapy
(2) Diagnosis of pregnancy
(3) Diagnosis of sexually transmitted diseases
(4) Prevention of immune rejection of organ implants
(5) Purification of industrial products
(6) Detection of trace molecules in food, agriculture and industry

The production of vaccines to combat human and animal diseases represents an immense market which has been extensively developed by the pharmaceutical industries. At present, vaccine quality and efficacy range from excellent to unsatisfactory.

In viral-derived diseases, vaccines are being developed by recombinant DNA technology against the influenza virus, polio virus, hepatitis B virus, herpes virus and, more recently, the AIDS virus. Successful vaccines in these important world diseases could mean massive commercial gains for the producing companies. The biggest opportunities exist for diseases such as AIDS or herpes where neither a vaccine nor a cure is yet available.

Extensive studies are also in progress with certain bacterial vaccines, as well as vaccines for parasitic diseases. Malaria still remains the most prevalent infectious disease in the world; this complex and demanding problem could well be overcome in the very near future.

A significant new development in medically related biotechnology has been the ability to produce monoclonal antibodies. A major advance of this technique is that, when antibody-producing cells are immortalised and stabilised, the secreted antibodies will always be the same from that particular cell line and can be fully characterised to assess their suitability for different applications. In this way suitable antibodies can be produced and scaled-up (either as ascites tumours in mice or by various forms of fermentation technology) in large quantities, allowing much greater standardisation for diagnostic applications. Monoclonal antibodies are now finding wide applications in diagnostic techniques that require highly specific reagents for the detection and measurement of soluble proteins and cell surface markers in blood transfusions, haematology, histology, microbiology and clinical chemistry, as well as in other non-medical areas (Table 8.2).

Monoclonals may also be used in the treatment of tumours, and possibly to carry cytotoxic drugs directly to the tumour site. In particular, monoclonals have found ready application in *in vitro* diagnostic products which do not need such rigorous safety testing. Diagnosis can be achieved for many diseases, including human venereal diseases, hepatitis B and some bacterial diseases. Monoclonals can also be used in pregnancy testing.

On a commercial scale, monoclonal antibodies are being produced in 100-litre airlift fermenters, by encapsulation in 100-litre fermenters, and in perfusion chambers using lymph from live cattle.

Commercially, monoclonals have been one of the most rewarding areas of new biotechnology. At present, immunoassays account for about 30% of total diagnostic testing sales and had achieved US$10 billion by the year 2000. In comparison, the DNA probe market for disease monitoring has expanded to about US$1.0 billion in the same time.

The twentieth century has witnessed tremendous advances in the diagnosis, understanding, prevention and cure of many infectious diseases. The success of global vaccination programmes and the discovery and development of antibiotics falsely induced microbiologists and clinicians to consider that microbial infections were conquered. That is no longer the case with the arrival of new diseases such as AIDS and BSE, and the rapid spread of antibiotic resistance, and diseases that were believed to be under control have re-emerged. As Louis Pasteur stated: 'Messieurs, ce sont les microbes qui avant le dernier mot'.

8.5   Biopharmaceuticals

The vast majority of pharmaceutical products are compounds derived either from synthetic chemical processes, from naturally occurring sources (plants, microorganisms), or from combinations of both. Such compounds are used to regulate essential bodily functions or to combat disease-causing microorganisms. Increasing attention is now being directed to the body's own regulatory molecules, which occur normally only in very small concentrations and which have, predominantly, defied modern methods of extraction or synthesis. Limited quantities of some of these compounds have historically been derived from organs of cadavers and from blood banks. Genetic engineering is now increasingly being recognised as a practical means of providing some of these scarce molecules in unrestricted quantities. In practice, this involves inserting the necessary human-derived gene constructs into suitable host microorganisms, which will produce the therapeutic protein (biopharmaceutical) in quantities related to the scale of operation. Not only is it now possible to produce these biopharmaceuticals in a form identical to that normally occurring in the human body, but also to design meaningful improvements in activity, stability or bioavailability. Such products will also be free of the dangerous

Table 8.3. Biopharmaceuticals approved for marketing between 1982 and 1992

Product	Broad approved medical use	Year of market introduction
Insulin	Diabetes	1982
Human growth hormone	Growth deficiency	1985
Interferon-α	Cancer, viral infections	1985
Anti-T-cell	Organ transplantation	1986
Hepatitis B vaccine	Hepatitis B prevention	1987
Tissue plasmogen activator	Cardiovascular disease	1987
Erythropoietin	Anaemia	1989
Interleukin-2	Cancer	1992
Coagulation factor VIII	Haemophilia A	1992
Interleukin-10	Prevention of thrombocytopenia	1997

From Bienz-Tadmor [1993] *Bio/Technology*, 168–71.

contaminants that have occasionally arisen from extraction of cadavers, e.g. the degenerative brain disease Creutzfeldt–Jakob disease has been associated with early human growth-hormone extractions.

The successful development of biopharmaceuticals requires:

(1) advanced biochemical/biomedical research to identify and characterise the native compounds;
(2) skilled molecular biology and cloning technology to identify the relevant gene sequences and insert them into a production mammalian or micro-biological host;
(3) bioprocess technology to grow the organisms and to isolate, concentrate and purify the chosen compounds;
(4) clinical and marketing expertise.

Table 8.3 indicates some of the main biopharmaceuticals approved for marketing worldwide between 1982 and mid-1992. It is probable that 50–100 new biopharmaceuticals are currently undergoing final clinical trials. The current worldwide market for biopharmaceuticals is well in excess of US$5 billion and is expected to approach $10 billion by 2020.

However, the use of these protein-type pharmaceuticals has several restrictions which will limit their use and size of market. As proteins, they are unstable and poorly absorbed from the gastrointestinal tract – consequently they have to be given parenterally by a medically trained person. Thus, their main use will be for acute, rather than chronic, conditions. Some proteins may also cause allergic reactions in the patient with long-term therapy.

A wide range of cellular forms, including bacteria, yeasts and mammalian and human cells, have been used for heterologous protein expression. Transgenic animals and plants can also be used as expression vehicles. When a transgene is introduced into a recipient animal, the expression of the gene product can occur in the milk, blood or urine of the animal.

With the advent of gene technology it is now possible to produce human therapeutic proteins in large quantities and of high purity. As such, recombinant human proteins can now be used in rational therapy using the body's own substances, which will not be immunogenic. To date, in excess of 60 recombinant proteins are now being used in therapy (Table 8.3), while over 200 others are in advanced development. It is anticipated that, in the near future, at least 100 pharmaceuticals derived from gene technology will be available for medical use. The DNA sequences coding for the therapeutic proteins can also be modified by direct mutagenesis, allowing further changes in protein structure. This is called '*protein engineering*' and the mutated proteins are termed '*muteins*'.

The first human gene sequences, encoding important therapeutic proteins, cloned into microorganisms were insulin, human growth hormone (somatostatin) and interferons.

Insulin

Throughout the world there are millions of people who need regular intakes of insulin to overcome the lethal effects of diabetes. Insulin extracted from pigs and cattle has long been the source of worldwide usage and it is now believed that some of the unfortunate side-effects that have occurred with continued long-term use of insulin could be due to additional contaminating compounds present in the animal insulin. Recombinant human insulin appears not to have such problems and is increasingly having the largest market share of sales. Production is unlimited and free from market shortage of animals and all the problems associated with previous production methods.

Somatostatin

The growth hormone somatostatin has been extremely difficult to isolate from animals; half a million sheep brains were required to be extracted to give 0.005 g of pure somatostatin. By cloning the human gene for somatostatin into a bacterium, this same amount of hormone can be produced from 9 litres of a transgenic bacterial fermentation. One child in 5000 suffers from hypopituitary dwarfism resulting from growth hormone deficiency and the easy availability of this biopharmaceutical will have immense benefit to these child sufferers. The annual world market is estimated at $100 million.

However, a potential massive market could arise from the increasing evidence that this growth hormone can increase muscle formation in normal individuals and is now being exploited by some athletes. There are also claims that regular administration of the hormone can improve quality of life in the aged!

Interferons

In 1957, two British researchers discovered substances produced within the body that could act against viruses by making cells resistant to virus attack. Most vertebrate animals can produce these substances, known as 'interferons', and many animal viruses can induce their *in vitro* synthesis and become sensitive to them. Why, then, have the interferons not become the 'penicillins' of virus infections? Primarily, this is because only minute amounts of interferon are produced within cells, and it has proved unbelievably complicated to extract and separate them from other cellular proteins.

Human interferons are glycoproteins (proteins with attached sugar molecules) and are believed to play a part in controlling many types of viral infections, including the common cold, as well as having potential in controlling cancer. However, the scarcity of these compounds has consistently hampered efforts to understand the extent of their effectiveness.

There are many different types of interferons, characteristic of individual species of animals; mouse interferons will respond to mouse cells but not to human cells, and vice versa. Furthermore, different tissues from the same species appear to produce different interferons. Thus, interferon for human studies must be derived from human cells, and it has been here that the blockage to production has occurred. Most early human interferon production was carried out in Finland using leucocyctes from blood, and the small amounts of interferon produced this way were used for limited clinical tests throughout the world.

So far, studies have shown that interferons can confer resistance to some virus infections and are involved in the body's natural immune reactions, even in the absence of viruses. However, much of the current interest in interferons arises from their ability to inhibit cancer in experimental animals.

Interferons present a new approach to cancer therapy because they appear to attack the cancer cells by inhibiting their growth, and that of any viruses involved in the cancer process, and they can also stimulate the body's natural immune defences against the cancer cell. Although the limited clinical studies of these compounds have indicated considerable potential in cancer therapy, the restricted supplies have severely hampered conclusive experimentation; this must await greater availability of interferons.

Two sources of interferon are currently available. The first source is from human diploid fibroblasts growing attached to a suitable surface, and the interferon produced is widely considered to be the safest available. The second source is from bacteria in which the gene for human fibroblast interferon has been inserted into a plasmid in such a manner that interferon is synthesised and can be extracted and purified.

Lymphokines

Lymphokines are proteins produced by lymphocytes (part of the body's immune system) and are considered to be crucially important to immune reactions. They appear to have the capability of enhancing or restoring the immune system to fight infectious diseases or cancer. Several lymphokines such as interleukin-2 at present offer great potential and are now produced by genetic engineering and are consequently more readily available on the market.

With each of these important compounds it has been possible to achieve a level of realistic pharmaceutical drug delivery only because recombinant DNA technology enabled the synthesis of large quantities of the product.

The production of human vaccines by recombinant methods has been quite successful and should allow for new approaches to diseases without existing remedial treatments. Recombinant hepatitis B virus has gained regulatory approval and has high market sales.

Presently, all biopharmaceuticals are produced by way of genetically engineered mammalian cell or microbial fermentations. However, with the development of transgenic animals (Chapter 10) it has become possible to produce certain human proteins of biopharmaceutical potential, including tissue plasmogen activator, blood clotting factors, etc., in the lactating glands of several animal species, such as mouse, sheep, cow and pig, and to be able to express the products in the milk of the animal. These products can then be more easily extracted and purified. A further feature of this process is that it is accomplished in a mammalian system which can confer on certain human proteins the complex structural modifications required for full biological activity. Such modifications cannot be achieved in microbial systems. As yet, no commercial production is in operation and it awaits improvements in yields and final regulatory approval. Undoubtedly this will become a major source of production of certain complex human proteins. There are no apparent adverse effects on the animal, which continues to produce milk in the normal way.

An American company can now produce human haemoglobin in the blood of transgenic pigs and, as such, this could serve as a human blood substitute. Such transgenic haemoglobin could capture a massive market. Each year worldwide, 70 million units of human blood are transfused at a cost of $10 billion. This transgenic haemoglobin would be free of human pathogens such as HIV and would not need typing or matching before transfusion because it is not composed of red blood cells. Much yet needs to be done before this becomes a reality.

Pharming – producing human pharmaceuticals in transgenic animals – is rapidly becoming a reality. The animals can be considered, in biotechnology terms, as bioreactors operating on a continuous basis. Overall this could be a massive worldwide market. At present the major limiting factor is achieving the number of transgenic animals, with the cost of producing such herds of animals being financially restrictive (Chapter 10).

8.6   Gene therapy

Undoubtedly, the most far reaching and controversial area of the genetic engineering of humans is gene therapy. Gene therapy can be considered as any treatment strategy that involves the introduction of genes or genetic material into human cells to alleviate or eliminate disease. The aim of gene therapy is to replace or repress defective genes with sequences of DNA that encode a specific genetic message. Within the cells, the DNA molecules may provide new genetic instructions to correct the host phenotype. However, to bring this about, the exogenous genes must first achieve passage to the disease cells. Herein lies the main and continuing difficulty. To date, gene therapy has been used to treat over 5000 people worldwide who suffer from a range of genetic disorders, but only a small number have shown clinical benefit. The majority of current gene therapy clinical trials involve the infective mechanisms of viruses, in particular retroviruses. These vectors are able to integrate, at random, sites in the host's cell genome and can pose risks to patients owing to random insertional mutagenesis and potential oncogenesis (cancer). Other approaches include direct injection of the gene into the cell, merging it into the cell with a

Table 8.4. Selected human genetic diseases for possible single-gene therapy

Disease	Target tissue	Incidence
Thalassaemia	Bone marrow	1 : 600 in some populations
Cystic fibrosis	Liver	1 : 500
Duchenne muscular dystrophy	Muscle/brain	1 : 300 males
Haemophilia A	Liver	1 : 6000 males
Haemophilia B	Fibroblasts	1 : 30000 males

From Johnson [1991] *Chemistry & Industry*, 644–666.

fat particle called a liposome, or with antibody-like proteins that can recognise the cell surface.

The liposomes are able to encapsulate DNA molecules and act as vectors in the delivery of therapeutic genes. Much research is now in progress to develop efficient *in vivo* gene delivery systems. As an alternative to gene delivery there is also an active alternative strategy of gene repair. The natural regulatory elements of genes are retained and segments of synthetic DNA and RNA, which will hopefully interact with malfunctioning genes and repair them, are delivered to cells.

It is, however, essential to distinguish between *germ-cell gene therapy* and *somatic-cell gene therapy*. In germ-cell gene therapy, changes are directed at the individual's genetic make-up, which can be passed onto the offspring. Ethics and practical wisdom ensure that this type of therapy will *not* be permitted in any country in the foreseeable future. In contrast, in somatic cell therapy, functioning genes are introduced into body cells which lack them. The effects of the therapy are confined to the person undergoing the treatment and are *not* passed onto the offspring. Because only somatic cells are receiving the human DNA, the treatment will probably have to be repeated for the person's lifetime.

The main thrust of gene therapy has been directed at correcting single-gene defects (mutations) which have been observed in families by their Mendelian pattern of inheritance, such as cystic fibrosis and haemophilia (Table 8.4). It is believed by some that many hundreds of such diseases could be treated by this process, and the next decade should see significant progress if the many technical problems can be readily overcome. At present, most genetic diseases have no effective treatment, so gene therapy could offer hope for so many people. Somatic-cell gene therapy for complex multifactorial diseases, e.g. Parkinson's disease and cancer, must be a long way off. In many of these

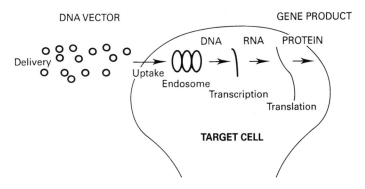

Fig. 8.3 Functional steps in gene transfer and expression. Gene therapy involves the delivery of DNA vectors to specific target cells within the body, uptake (commonly by endocytosis), transcription and translation of sequences within the DNA vector, and production of a therapeutic gene product.

diseases there can be many genes involved as well as an interaction with environmental factors.

Gene therapy has not yet lived up to its original promise, but some recent successes in the treatment of certain genetic blood diseases may herald a new era of success. The potential of this area of medical science could yet be realised in the near future.

Gene therapy is a complex series of events relying heavily on new biotechnological techniques. Therapy will require a full understanding both of the mechanism by which the defective or unusual gene exerts its effect on the individual, and of the ability to switch off the defective gene and substitute a healthy gene copy (Fig. 8.3). It is truly a multidisciplinary activity involving skills in molecular biology, cell biology, virology, pharmacology, clinical application and patient interaction. The USA are the undoubted world leaders in gene-therapy research and application. Some of the protocols are now proceeding through regulatory processes, and already patent coverage for gene construction, delivery systems and supporting technology has been granted. Private medical systems internationally must view gene therapy as a very lucrative market in the affluent nations.

8.7 A cautionary note

The latter years of the twentieth century will be remembered for the remarkable advances that have been made in molecular genetics, with the elucidation of the human genome as the major achievement. Accompanying these outstanding discoveries, the reductionist biomedical community has been consistently propounding exaggerated claims about how these scientific discoveries were going to revolutionise medical treatments. By contrast, achievements in molecular medicine have been quite limited. While medical biotechnology has been heavily investing in genome-based research, on the assumption that the complexities of cell function in health and disease could be unravelled using knowledge of genes alone, there has been insufficient emphasis *and funding* on other aspects of cellular organisation. It is now clear that cellular organisation is not simply a projection of the organisation of the genome; rather, there is a complex myriad of control and signalling pathways that must be coordinated at cellular, tissue and whole-organism level. Even diseases resulting from single-gene mutation can have complex pathogenesis. For most diseases, there will be large numbers of genes and environmental factors contributing to their aetiology, making a molecular explanation decidedly impossible.

Molecular scientists are now concentrating much of their efforts on proteomics since most of the control-circuit components in health and disease occur at the protein level. Proteomics is now being used to identify and compare complex protein profiles, which could lead to generating sensitive molecular fingerprints of proteins that are present in body fluids at a particular time and in specific diseases. The first major medical use of these studies could be early diagnosis of many diseases, possibly allowing earlier treatment protocols to be started. However, it must be said that it could be many years, if not decades, before molecular biology realises many medical successes.

While the current strategies are increasingly producing a wealth of information on the molecular composition and structure at the cellular level, this is not reflected at whole-organ and whole-body level. It must also be said that the reductionist molecular biology approach now pervades teaching programmes in most biological subjects, to their detriment. It is important that science should be seen to benefit society and it is perhaps time that grant funding bodies assessed the long-term relevance of molecular biology to the nation's health. A vast proportion of national health research budgets is directed to molecular aspects of genomics and proteomics, which will undoubtedly produce a wealth of scientific knowledge, but will it lead to a huge advancement in applicable medical practice?

9

Environmental biotechnology

9.1 Introduction

As societies throughout the world are increasingly moving to greater levels of urbanisation and industrial development, public concern is mounting over the state of the environment, and much attention is now being given to improving the environment for future generations. To achieve this, there has been, particularly in developed nations, major environmental legislation directed towards liquid, solid and hazardous wastes. In most developing countries the situation is less encouraging, where financing is limited, or not available, for the construction of water and waste-treatment facilities and where there is a shortage of trained personnel to operate the systems. Furthermore, in many developing countries there is a lack of official regulations and control systems, no administration bodies responsible for waste control, and little obligation for existing and emerging industries to dispose of waste properly. Also, it is in such countries that there is the greatest movement towards urbanisation and new industrial development, with concomitant destruction of the environment.

Waste generation is a side-effect of consumption and production activities, and tends to rise with the level of economic advance. Wastes arise from domestic and industrial activity, e.g. sewage, waste waters, agriculture and food wastes from processing, wood wastes, and an ever-increasing range of toxic industrial chemical products and by-products. In the final assessment, wastes represent the end of the technical and economic life of products. Costs for properly dealing with wastes are escalating and much attention is presently devoted to efficient and effective waste management, which will include costs of collection, storage, processing and removal of wastes.

Probably the most disturbing aspect of pollution is the increasing presence of toxic chemicals in the natural environment. The large-scale production and application of synthetic chemicals and their subsequent pollution of the environment is now a problem of serious concern in most industrialised countries and must be viewed as an extreme threat to the self-regulating capacity of the biosphere in which we live. The US Environmental Protection Agency's list of high-awareness pollutants includes most pesticides, halogenated aliphatics, aromatics, polychlorinated biphenyls, polycyclic aromatic hydrocarbons and nitrosamines.

While many of these compounds are used directly by man in agriculture and public health for obvious and beneficial results, others may be derived from a spectrum of industrial processes that are used to make a variety of useful products. Some are associated with the petroleum industry and others are solvents. Such toxic and hazardous chemicals are insidiously entering a variety of environments. These synthetic compounds can be found at very high concentrations at the point of discharge, such as factory sites and industrial spillages, where they can exert pronounced deleterious effects, while others occur at low levels in natural environments but because of their inherent toxicity, e.g. the pesticide dioxin, they constitute a serious health hazard.

In many parts of the world there is increasing evidence that underground water sources are demonstrating dangerous levels of contamination. In continental Europe a notorious example of such industrially derived pollution is the valley of the River Po in North Italy, where there has been permanent abandonment of groundwater sources. Similar examples occur in parts of the Netherlands lying below the level of the notoriously polluted river Rhine. Such chemical pollutants can remain in water-bearing rocks for decades and measures of removal would be lengthy, unbelievably complicated and restrictively costly.

It is now clear that many past and present industrial products and processes can be seen as environmentally unfriendly and are major sources of pollution. Historically, civil engineering or, more specifically, sanitary engineering dealt mechanistically with such socially important areas as drinking water, catchment and treatment, waste water (domestic and industrial), solid wastes and industrial off-gases. The bio-component of all these processes was largely ignored. While biotechnological processes have always been part of these industrial activities, they are now increasingly being viewed in an overall environmental context. Environmental biotechnology is the application of recognised biotechnology processes towards the protection and restoration of the quality of the environment, especially with a long-term perspective.

While industrial biotechnology largely utilises known microorganisms in product formation, environmental biotechnology will mainly rely on microbial consortia of complex and variable composition. New studies are now identifying and characterising the microorganisms which exist and interact in soils, in anaerobic systems and in domestic and industrial waste streams. Can such mixed-culture systems accept new improved microorganisms, and what will be the regulatory constraints on the deliberate introduction of modified microorganisms into the environment? The potential to enhance the degradative potential of microorganisms to degrade recalcitrant pollutants is immense and must be examined cautiously but creatively. Rehabilitation of contaminated land and waters is a major task for present and future generations. Of equal importance is the need to prevent future contamination from ongoing manufacturing processes, namely clean technology.

9.2   Microbial ecology/environmental biotechnology

The presence and functioning of microbial communities affect our everyday lives in so many ways, but none more so than their role in soil, waste and water management. Historically, the need to supply populations with safe drinking water and acceptable sewage disposal has mainly been the concern of sanitary engineers. (Engineering-driven solutions to these basic sanitary problems of communities were evolving long before there was any appreciation of the intrinsic roles of microorganisms.) More recently, the skills and knowledge of the microbiologist are increasingly being employed to develop new systems.

Microbial ecology is the science that studies the interrelationships between microorganisms and their living (biotic) and non-living (abiotic) environments. The increasing scientific and public awareness of microbial ecology since the 1960s derives mainly from the recognition of the central role of microorganisms in maintaining good environmental quality. It is the microbes in their multivarious forms that largely direct the orderly flow of materials and energy (biogeochemical cycles) through the world's ecosystems by way of their immense and varied metabolic abilities to transform inorganic and organic materials. Microbial ecology is an extremely relevant scientific discipline with proven practical applications and must be viewed as one of the most critical scientific approaches to environmental problems.

Biodegradation can be defined as the decomposition of substances by microbial activities either by single organisms or, most often, by microbial consortia. Microorganisms found in soil and water will attempt to utilise any organic substances encountered as sources of energy and carbon by enzymatically

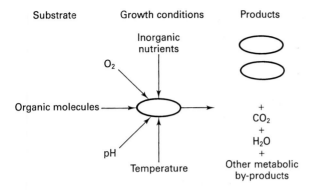

Fig. 9.1   Natural microbial biodegradation of organic molecules.

breaking them down into simple molecules that can be absorbed and used. Under suitable environmental conditions, all natural organic compounds should be degraded (Fig. 9.1) and, for this reason, large-scale deposits of naturally formed organic compounds are rarely observed. When such organic deposits do occur, e.g. coal and oil, it has been under conditions that are hostile to biodegradation.

Environmental biotechnology will include the application of biological systems and processes in waste treatment and management. Many successful biotechnological processes have now been developed for water, gas, soil and solid waste treatments. Modern developments in environmental biotechnology now focus on process optimisation and will no longer accept processes which are inefficient and which sometimes merely transform one problem into another, e.g. formation of carcinogenic nitrosamine compounds by the reaction of some microorganisms with organic amines and nitrous oxide. Environmental safety should not be threatened by environmental processes.

Organic chemicals that cannot easily be degraded by microorganisms, or are indeed totally resistant to attack, are termed 'recalcitrant', e.g. lignin. Xenobiotics are man-made synthetic compounds not formed by natural biosynthetic processes and, in many cases, can be recalcitrant. A xenobiotic compound is, therefore, a foreign substance in our ecosystem and may often have toxic effects. All environmental biotechnological processes make use of the metabolic (degradative and anabolic) activities of microorganisms, demonstrating, again, the indispensable nature of microbes in our ecosystem.

The term 'biodegradable' is often loosely identified with the term 'environmentally friendly', and numerous advertising campaigns and product packaging have put across the message that, because a product is biodegradable, its impact on the environment will be dramatically reduced. This is not always the case, and demonstrations of product biodegradability have often only been achieved under highly conducive microbial conditions that are not easily met in the natural environment. Furthermore, biodegradability itself is a complex multifactorial event whose mechanisms are not completely understood. A range of environmental waste-treatment technologies will now be examined.

9.3   Waste-water and sewage treatment

While many ancient civilisations had an appreciation of the need to protect the quality of water to be used for human consumption, it was not until 1855 that it was demonstrated that cholera was transmitted by water contaminated with faeces. A similar route for typhoid fever was shortly to be demonstrated. By the end of the nineteenth century, the microbial ecology of many human diseases had been shown to have an anal–oral route of transmission, which finally confirmed the health hazards associated with water contaminated with faeces. The introduction of sewage systems in developed societies during the nineteenth century allowed, for the first time, the possibility of treatment of municipal and industrial wastes before discharge into natural water systems.

Growth in human populations has generally been matched by a concomitant formation of a wider range of waste products, many of which cause serious environmental pollution if they are allowed to accumulate in the ecosystem. In rural communities, recycling of human, animal and vegetable wastes has been practised for centuries, providing in many cases valuable fertilisers or fuel. However, it was also a source of disease to humans and animals by residual pathogenicity of enteric (intestinal) bacteria. In urban communities, where most of the deleterious wastes accumulate, efficient waste collection and specific treatment processes have been developed, since it is impractical to discharge high volumes of waste into natural land and waters. The introduction of these practices in the last century was one of the main reasons for the spectacular improvement in health and well-being in the developed countries.

Mainly by empirical means, a variety of biological treatment systems have been developed, ranging from cesspits, septic tanks and sewage farms to gravel beds, percolating filters and activated sludge processes coupled with anaerobic digestion. The primary aims of all of these systems or bioreactors is to alleviate health hazards and to reduce the amount of biologically oxidisable organic compounds, producing a final effluent or outflow that can be discharged into the natural environment without any adverse effects.

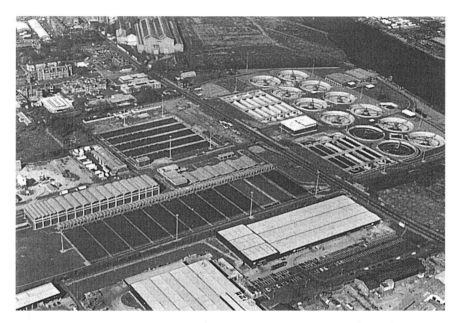

Fig. 9.2   Aerial view of bioreactors at the sewage treatment plant for the city of Glasgow, Scotland.

Such bioreactor assemblies rely on the metabolic versatility of mixed microbial populations (microbial ecology) for their efficiency. The systems in which they perform their biological functions can be likened to other industrial bioreactors (e.g. as in antibiotic production); large-scale plants, e.g. municipal forced-aeration tanks (Fig. 9.2), can be extremely complex, requiring the skills of the engineer and the microbiologist for successful operation. The fundamental feature of these bioreactors is that they contain a range of microorganisms with the overall metabolic capacity to degrade most organic compounds entering the system.

The development of these systems was an early example of biotechnology. Indeed, in volumetric terms, biological treatment of domestic waste-waters and sewerage in the industrialised nations is by far the largest biotechnological industry and the least recognised by lay people. Controlled use of microorganisms has led to the virtual elimination of such waterborne diseases as typhoid, cholera and dysentery in these communities. Yet, if water and sewage treatments are seriously interrupted, major epidemics may quickly develop, as witnessed in 1968 in Zermatt, Switzerland, where typhoid developed following the breakdown of the water treatment plant.

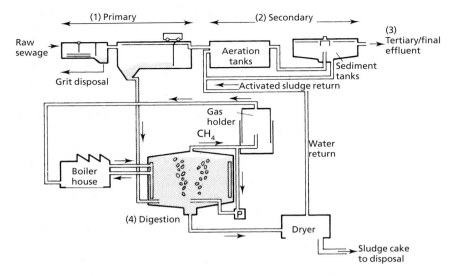

Fig. 9.3   Stages of sewage treatment in a complex incorporating anaerobic digestion.

Thus, biotechnology not only generates a whole new range of useful products, it also plays an indispensable part – through water- and sewage-treatment processes – in the reduction of infectious diseases of humans and animals.

The biological disposal of organic wastes is achieved in many ways throughout the world. A widely used practice for sewage treatment is shown in Fig. 9.3. This complex but highly successful system involves a series of three stages of primary and secondary processing followed by microbial digestion. An optional tertiary stage involving chemical precipitation may be included. The primary activity is to remove coarse particles and solubles, leaving the dissolved organic materials to be degraded or oxidised by microorganisms in a highly aerated, open bioreactor. This secondary process requires considerable energy input to drive the mechanical aerators that actively mix the whole system, ensuring regular contact of the microorganisms with the substrates and air. The microorganisms multiply and form a biomass or sludge, which can either be removed and dumped, or passed to an anaerobic digester (bioreactor) which will reduce the volume of solids, the odour and the number of pathogenic microorganisms. A further useful feature is the generation of methane or biogas, which can be used as a fuel. However, the value of biogas is marginal because of its content of carbon dioxide and hydrogen sulphide.

Another important means of degrading dilute organic liquid wastes is the percolating or trickling filter bioreactor. In this system the liquid flows over a series of surfaces, which may be stones, gravel, plastic sheets, etc., on which attached microbes remove organic matter for essential growth. Excessive microbial growth can be a problem, creating blockages and loss of biological activity. Such techniques are widely used in water purification systems.

Abundant availability of water is vital for modern urban and industrial development. Water makes up more than 70% of the human body and about 2 litres per day is usually sufficient to keep an adult healthy. Water acts as a transport medium for essential nutrients within the body, helps to remove toxins and waste materials, stabilises the body temperature and performs a crucial part in the structure and function of the circulatory system. *In essence, water is the elixir of life.* In the natural world the ecosystem regenerates and recycles water. Increasingly, man's intrusion into nature by industrialisation, extensive farming practices, deforestation, etc., has severely unbalanced this process. It is now accepted that two-thirds of the world's nations are water-stressed – using clean water faster than it is replenished in aquifers or rivers. Biotechnology will play an important role in reclamation and purification of waste waters for re-use. Water must be recycled in the sustainable use of resources. The most important threat mankind faces in the coming decades is not global warming or energy deficiency but an increasing shortage of high-quality water.

What are the future areas of importance? Microbiological effluent treatment will be a major field of biotechnological interest in the future. Integrated systems will be developed for treating complex wastes. The role of the biocatalyst or microbe will be constantly reassessed.

In countries with high annual hours of sunlight, there has been considerable development of combined algal/bacterial systems for waste and water treatments. Such processes can lead to the formation of relatively pure water and algal/bacterial biomass, which may be used for animal feeding, for biogas formation or, perhaps more ambitiously, for bulk organic chemical formation.

A novel biotechnological innovation in waste-water treatment is the deep-shaft fermentation system developed by ICI. The deep shaft is, in fact, a hole in the ground (up to 150 metres in depth), divided to allow the cycling and mixing of waste water, air and microorganisms (Fig. 9.4). It is most economical in land use and power, and produces much less sludge than conventional systems.

A comparison of several widely used treatment processes for liquid wastes is shown in Table 9.1.

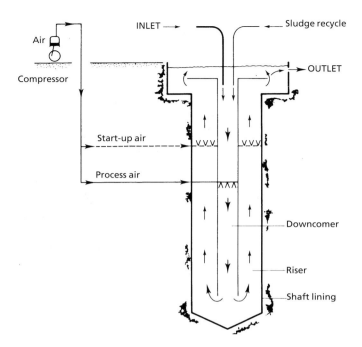

Fig. 9.4 The principle of the deep-shaft fermentation system used in waste-water treatment.

9.4 Landfill technologies

Solid wastes account for an increasing proportion of the waste streams generated by modern urban societies. While part of this material will be made up of glass, plastics, etc., a considerable proportion will be decomposable solid organic material, such as paper, food wastes, sewage wastes, wastes from large-scale poultry and pig farms, and, in the USA in particular, cattle feed lot wastes.

In large urbanised communities, the essential disposal of such wastes is problematic, and one well-used system is by low-cost anaerobic landfill technology. In this procedure solid wastes are deposited in low-lying, low-value sites and each day's waste deposit is compressed and covered by a layer of soil. The complete filling of such sites can take months or years, depending on size of site and flow of wastes. They can be unsightly, smelly and unhygienic if improperly managed. Also, toxic wastes can create severe problems for the microbiological process occurring in the site, together with toxic run-off.

Table 9.1. Comparison of aerobic biological treatment processes for liquid wastes

Process	Advantages	Disadvantages
Aerated lagoons	High BOD* removal efficiency Low operating costs Requires low-skilled operators	Can foul-up and create smells Solids carry-over Considerable land requirements Sensitive to cold weather
Activated sludge	High BOD removal efficiency Moderate ground requirements	High energy consumptions Requires disposal of excess sludge Requires skilled operators Sensitive to sudden high inputs
Trickling filters	Low operator costs Moderate space requirements Resistant to sudden high inputs	Moderate BOD removal Disposal of excess sludge necessary
Rotating biological contactors	High BOD removal efficiency Compact Moderate energy input	Possible odour formation Requires skilled operators Disposal of excess sludge required

* BOD, biological oxygen demand – the amount of dissolved oxygen required by aerobic microorganisms to stabilise organic matter in waste water or sludge; sludge, microbial aggregates or flocs that can be separated from the purified effluent via sedimentation.

Improperly prepared and operated landfill sites may result in toxic heavy metals, hazardous pollutants and products of anaerobic decomposition seeping from the site into underground aquifers and subsequently polluting urban water supplies. Properly constructed and sealed landfill sites (Fig. 9.5) can be used to generate methane gas, for commercial use. Much effort is now made to use strong, impermeable liners to avoid leachates damaging surrounding land and water courses.

Current regulations require new landfill sites to be air- and water-tight to protect the environment. Regular monitoring is necessary to detect contamination of groundwater, surface water and surrounding air. Landfill owners

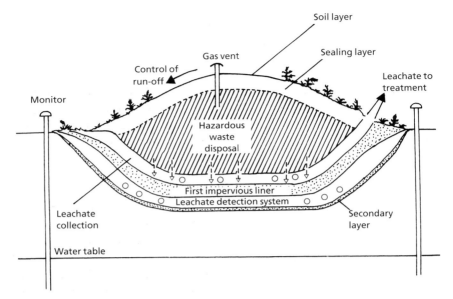

Fig. 9.5   A landfill site that conforms to new regulations.

are now *financially* responsible for the long-term care of the sites *after* final closure. Landfill operations should be viewed as gigantic bioreactors, with methane as the usable product. Methane production will usually commence several months after proper construction and filling of the site, proceeding through a peak production period and gradually declining after a number of years.

In the past, landfill sites were seen essentially as 'dumping' sites or storage vessels where the waste was essentially sealed from the surrounding environment. Nowadays, in sharp contrast, new sites are managed as bioreactor vessels where correct stabilisation-enhancement systems are operated during the working life of the landfill site. Current practice in most western nations is to reduce the amount of waste to be landfilled and to increase the safety of the operation. However, the practice of landfilling will continue to have an important role in the overall management of solid wastes in the foreseeable future.

9.5   Composting

Composting is an aerobic, microbial-driven process that converts solid organic wastes into a stable, sanitary, humus-like material which has been considerably reduced in bulk and which can be safely returned to the environment. It is, in effect, a low-moisture, solid-substrate fermentation process, as previously discussed (Chapter 4). To be totally effective, it should only use as substrates readily decomposable solid organic waste. In large-scale operations using largely domestic solid organic wastes, the final product is mostly used for soil improvement, but in more specialised operations using specific organic raw substrates (straw, animal manures, etc.), the final product can become the substrate for the worldwide commercial production of the mushroom *Agaricus bisporus*.

Composting has long been recognised not only as a means of safely treating solid organic wastes but particularly as a form of recycling of organic matter. Composting will increasingly play a significant role in future waste management schemes since it offers the means of re-use of organic material derived from domestic, agriculture and food industry wastes. The increased interest in composting derives from the growing awareness of the many environmental problems associated with some of the main ways now practised for treating solid organic wastes, e.g. incineration and landfilling. The overwhelming majority of municipalities and individuals are opposed to having incinerators and landfill sites established within their communities.

Composting has only recently become a serious waste-management technology, and both theoretical and practical development of the technology is still in its infancy. The primary aim of a composting operation is to obtain, in a limited time within a limited compost, a final compost with a desired product quality. A composting plant must function under environmentally safe conditions.

Composting is carried out in a packed bed of solid organic particles in which the indigenous microbes will grow and reproduce. Free access to air is an essential requirement. The starting materials are arranged in static piles (windrows), aerated piles or covered tunnels or in rotating bioreactors (drums or cylinders). Some form of pre-treatment of the waste may be required, such as particle-size reduction by shredding or grinding. The basic biological reaction of the composting process is the oxidation of the mixed organic substrates with oxygen to produce carbon dioxide, water and other organic by-products (Fig. 9.6). After the composting process is completed, the final product most often needs to be left for variable time periods to stabilise.

Successful composting requires optimisation of the growth conditions for the microorganisms. It is a mixed-culture fermentation and an outstanding example of microbial ecology in action. The large bulk of most operations acts as insulation and, as a result of the biological heat generated by the microbial reactions, there can be rapid internal heat build-up. Over-heating can seriously

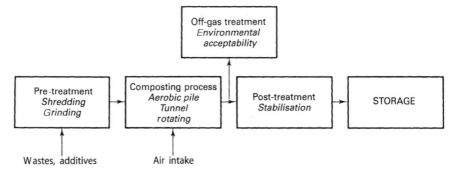

Fig. 9.6 Flow chart for composting plant process.

impair microbial activity. Compost processes should be regulated to prevent temperature rising above 55°C. The moisture level of the organic substrates should normally be 45–60%; above 60%, free moisture will accumulate, filling the interparticle spaces and restricting aeration, while below 40%, conditions become too dry for successful microbial colonisation.

Solid organic materials are only slowly solubilised by exo-enzyme secretion by the fermenting microbes. This reaction step is generally considered as rate-limiting. Cellulose and lignin are abundantly present in most solid wastes. A high lignin content, for example, in straw and wood materials, hampers the overall process of degradation. Lignin is especially resistant to degradation and is only slowly degraded. In many instances it can shield other substances which are otherwise more easily degraded. Ready access to air is an essential ingredient for a successful, balanced bioreactor.

For large-scale commercial composting, the aerated pile system is carried out in closed buildings to facilitate the control of odour emissions. In these systems forced aeration with regular turning is used to create good composting conditions. There are now several plants in Europe with a capacity of over 60 000 tonnes per year.

Tunnel composting is performed in closed plastic tunnels 30–50 m long and 4–6 m in width and height. Such tunnel systems have been in operation for many years for the composting of sewage sludge and domestic wastes and for specialised substrate preparation for mushroom production. Some plants can operate at up to 10 000 tonnes per year.

Rotating drum systems in various sizes have been used for composting domestic wastes worldwide. The large Dano process is especially useful for wettish organic waste. Small drum systems have been widely accepted for small quantities of garden waste which can readily be used for recycling.

In some composting processes the waste gas outlets can create odour problems owing to the presence of sulphur and nitrogen compounds. Special attention is now given to reducing or removing these odours by gas scrubbers or filtration since environmental regulations can lead to the closure of offending plants. The most widely used form of biofiltration involves a fixed bed or mass of organic material, e.g. mature compost or microbially embedded wood chips. The gases pass through the mixture and the resulting biochemical activity can greatly reduce the offensive chemical smells.

Composting is undoubtedly one of the principal strategies for solid organic waste treatment and recycling back into the environment.

For future expansion of composting and recycling, four criteria will need to be achieved:

(1) a suitable infrastructure must be in place;
(2) suitable quality and quantity of substrates must be available;
(3) there must be markets for the end-products;
(4) processes must be environmentally sound and demonstrate economic viability.

In 1992, 7% of all European municipal solid waste was composted and, by 2000, this had grown to almost 18%. Germany, as a renowned 'green' nation, already has a much higher rate. During 1992, no less than 120 composting plants were being built, enlarged or planned in Germany. This would add a compost production capacity of nearly 1 million tonnes annually.

A major reason for this expansion has been the separation of domestic waste at source. This is the three-bin approach widely practised in Europe, namely one for recyclables (glass, metals, plastics), one for fully degradables (vegetable wastes, papers – the bio-bin), and one for other materials and hazardous wastes.

In Germany alone it has been calculated that an annual demand for 20 million tonnes (MT) of compost can be identified, thus:

10.8 MT – agriculture

1.2 MT – viniculture

1 MT   – forestry

3.6 MT – substrates and soils

3.4 MT – land reclamation

The process of composting has been with us in many forms for centuries, recycling vegetable wastes into useful products. It is simple, natural and invariably costs less than landfill and incineration. But above all, it is safe, free from toxic emissions, and needs minimum financial resources.

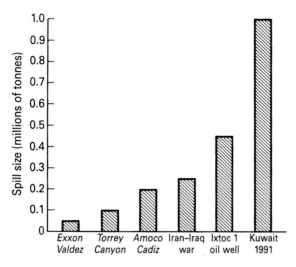

Fig. 9.7   Estimated size of major oil spills.

9.6   Bioremediation

Large areas of the earth's surfaces and the oceans and other waterways have already been contaminated with oil-derived compounds and toxic chemicals. More than two million tonnes of oil are estimated to enter the sea each year. Approximately half will be derived from industrial effluents, sewage and river outflows and the remainder from non-tanker shipping and natural seepage from below the seafloor. It is considered that only about 18% of the total is coming from refineries, off-shore operation and tanker activities. Unlike most other pollutants, oil spillages can readily be seen and have become an emotive subject on the TV screen. Most oils do have a relatively low toxicity to the environment in general but can have catastrophic and immediate effects on bird and animal life associated with water. Some of the major oil spills of recent years are shown in Fig. 9.7.

The contamination of soil normally results from a range of activities related to our industrialised society. Contaminated land is viewed as land that contains substances which, when present in sufficient quantities or concentrations, can probably cause harm to man – directly or indirectly – and to the environment in general. Many xenobiotic (industrially derived) compounds can show high levels of recalcitrance and, while in many cases only small concentrations get into the environment, they can be subject to biomagnification. Biomagnification, in essence, implies an increase in the concentration of a chemical substance, e.g. DDT, as the substance is passed through the food chain.

Hazardous wastes and chemicals have become one of the major problems of modern society worldwide. In the USA, in excess of 50 000 contaminated sites and several hundred thousand leaking underground storage tanks have been identified. The estimated cost of treating these polluted sites is 1.7×10^{12} and, to date, the US Environmental Pollution Agency (EPA) has given 15.2×10^9 to clean up hazardous waste sites. Hazardous wastes and toxic chemicals pose complex environmental problems by directly affecting the air, water, soil and sediments while indirectly and unpredictably affecting living organisms that use these resources.

The commitment of biotechnology for the environmental management of such hazardous wastes or contaminants can be seen as the development of systems that involve biological catalysts to degrade, detoxify or accumulate contaminating chemicals. The application of biological agents – mostly microorganisms – for the treatment of environmental chemicals has mostly been directed towards remedial activities.

There are three main approaches to be assessed in dealing with contaminated sites, namely: (1) identification; (2) assessment of the nature and degree of the hazard, and (3) the choice of remedial action.

When dealing with contaminated soil, clean-up operations can involve on-site processing, *in situ* treatment or off-site processing. Up to the present, a considerable degree of remedial activities have centred on physical and chemical methods of separation and/or removal of the pollutants. Such methods will not be further discussed in the present context but, rather, attention will be devoted to the increasingly used biological methods of remediation that are variously termed '*bioremediation*', '*bio-restoration*', '*bioreclamation*' or '*biotreatment*'.

The basic principles of bioremediation are superficially simple: optimise the environmental conditions so that microbial biodegradation can occur rapidly and as completely as possible. Microbes that are naturally present in soils and water environments are potential candidates for the biological transformation of xenobiotic compounds that are introduced into the ecosystem. Microbial populations in natural environments exist in a dynamic equilibrium that can be altered by modifying the environmental conditions, such as nutrient availability.

In almost all cases it will not be individual strains but consortia of microorganisms that will act on pollutant molecules. The metabolic effect of microorganisms on pollutants can take many forms and is not always to the environmental advantage of the ecosystems (Table 9.2).

Table 9.2. The effect of microbes on chemical pollutants

Category	Chemical change
Degradation	Complex compound transformed into simple products, sometimes mineralisation
Conjugation	Formation of complex or addition reactions to more complex compounds
Detoxification	Conversion to non-toxic compound(s)
Activation	Compound converted into more toxic compound

The application of bioremediation to environmental clean-up has been applied in two ways:

(1) Promotion of microbial growth *in situ* can be achieved by the addition of nutrients. When the indigenous microbial population has been exposed to specific polluting compounds for prolonged periods, subpopulations will have developed a limited metabolic ability to use, and thus degrade, the offending pollutant. However, growth of these particular microbes will invariably be nutrient-limited and, when essential growth nutrients such as nitrogen and phosphorus are added, growth stimulation will normally occur with a concomitant increase in pollutant breakdown. This method was successfully applied to beaches along Prince William Sound and the Gulf of Alaska in 1989/90 to clean up the oil spillage from the oil tanker Exxon Valdez. Fertilisers (nutrients), when applied in various formulations to the beaches, stimulated the indigenous microorganisms to degrade the oil to less harmful products, which subsequently became part of the food chain. Over three million dollars were spent on the bioremediation of the Alaskan beaches and, to date, has been the largest application of this emerging technology. Soils contaminated with recalcitrant chemicals such as polychlorinated biphenols (PCBs) – previously considered to be highly toxic and indestructible industrial pollutants – are now being realistically dechlorinated by this method.

(2) The alternative approach to direct nutrient supplementation and *in situ* microbial growth stimulation has been to remove microbial samples from the polluted site, enrich the useful microbes, scale-up from the mixture by bioreactor cultivation, and re-inoculate large quantities of the 'cocktail' of microbes into the contaminated site. This has been quite successful in some sites.

Some companies now market microbial inocula, which are claimed to significantly increase the rate of biodegradation of oil pollutants. Another approach has been to utilise and market white-rot fungi such as *Phanaerochytae chrysosporium*, a widely used degrader of lignocellulosic materials. Organisms that can degrade such complex organic molecules, e.g. lignin, have a wide range of enzymic activities which are capable of degrading many of the most dangerous industrial pollutants, e.g. PCBs. There are presently some constraints on this approach, *viz*:

(1) Indigenous degradative microbes are fully adapted to the specific environment to be treated.
(2) Introduced or 'foreign' microbes must be able to survive in the new environment and be able to compete with the established indigenous microbes.
(3) Added inocula must remain in close contact with the pollutant and, in aqueous environments, avoid dilution.

A further possibility in bioremediation is to genetically engineer microorganisms to be able to degrade those organic pollutant molecules that, at present they are unable to do. While this has been achieved in some cases, there are considerable technical problems, including genetic stability and survival of the 'new' microbe in a hostile environment. Furthermore, there are legislative, ethical and perceptional problems concerned with their release into environments such as sewage systems, soils and oceans. To date no genetically engineered microorganism has left the laboratory and been tested in the field. There is intense research in progress worldwide, particularly the USA, and it is believed by many informed industrial scientists that in the near future this technology may be widely and safely used for environmental applications.

The detection and disarming of land mines – a problem of huge dimensions in countries devastated by war – may well, in part, have a biotechnological amelioration. For example, certain microorganisms can utilise explosives such as 2,4,6 trinitrotoluene (TNT) as nutrient, and soil contaminated with TNT can be bioremediated. Since longstanding land mines invariably leak explosives into the near environment, it has been shown that, by inserting a gene for luminescence or fluorescence near the digestive enzyme, the bacteria would glow, thus enhancing recognition of the mine. This process exemplifies the bringing together of biosensor technology and bioremediation.

While microorganisms have dominated bioremediation practices, there is a groundswell of interest in using plants to remediate some environmental problems. Plants have evolved an exquisite root system that allows efficient acquisition of essential elements from soil. Removing from soil inorganic

Table 9.3. Strengths and weaknesses of bioremediation of oils

Strengths	Weaknesses
Relatively simple techniques	Can be slow when compared with physical clean-up methods.
Relatively low cost	Applicable only in certain environments and for compounds suitably biodegradable
Results in mineralisation or easily dispersed by-products	Involves addition of man-made chemicals/nutrients and dispersants – possible source of environmental contamination
Technology can be unobtrusive and non-disruptive	Requires explanation to the public regulators and bodies involved in environmental clean-up because it is a new technology
Accelerated natural biological mechanics avoid associated risks of man-made hazardous wastes	

From P. Morgan, Shell International Petroleum Co. Ltd, London.

pollutants such as lead, mercury and cadmium could well be a new, potentially low-cost, environmentally sound remediation strategy.

Bioremediation is a new technology and will require time for full development and application. Some of the relative strengths and weaknesses of bioremediation for the treatment of oil spillages are shown in Table 9.3.

9.7   Detection and monitoring of pollutants

A wide range of traditional methods have long been used to detect pollutants, including microbial and chemical analyses. More recently improved biological detection methods include biosensors and immunoassays. Such sensors can be designed to be highly selective or sensitive to a wide range of compounds, e.g. pesticides. Microbial biosensors are microorganisms which produce a reaction (such as luminescence light) upon contact with the substance to be sensed.

Immunoassays use labelled antibodies and enzymes to measure pollutant levels. Such assays have proved very valuable for sensitive and rapid field use. Another increasingly used technique for microbial detection is direct isolation and amplification of DNA from soil.

9.8   Microbes and the geological environment

Microbes are increasingly recognised as important catalytic agents in certain geological processes, e.g. mineral formation, mineral degradation, sedimentation, weathering and geochemical cycling.

One of the most detrimental examples of microbal involvement with minerals occurs in the production of acid mine waters. This occurs from microbial pyrite oxidation when bituminous coal seams are exposed to air and moisture during mining. In many mining communities, the huge volumes of sulphuric acid produced in this way have created pollution on an unprecedented scale. Other examples of the detrimental effects of microbes include the microbial weathering of building stone such as limestone, leading to defacement or structural changes.

In contrast to these harmful effects, microbes are increasingly used beneficially to extract commercially important elements by solubilisation (*bioleaching*). For example, metals like cobalt, copper, zinc, lead or uranium can be more easily separated from low-grade ores using microbial agents – mining with microbes.

The biological reactions in extractive metal leaching are usually concerned with the oxidation of mineral sulphides. Many bacteria, fungi, yeasts, algae and even protozoa are able to carry out these specific reactions. Many minerals exist in close association with other substances, e.g. sulphur, and iron sulphide, which must be oxidised to free the valuable metal. A widely used bacterium *Thiobacillus ferrooxidans* can oxidise both sulphur and iron, the sulphur in the ore wastes being converted by the bacteria to sulphuric acid. Simultaneously, the oxidation of iron sulphide to iron sulphate is enhanced.

The commercial process involves the repeated washing of crushed ore (normally in large heaps, Fig. 9.8) with a bioleaching solution containing live microorganisms and some essential nutrients (phosphate/ammonia) to encourage their growth. The leach liquor collected from the heaps contains the essential metal, which can easily be separated (downstream processing) by sulphuric acid extraction.

In the USA, almost 10% of total copper production is obtained by this method. Countries such as India, Canada, the USA, Chile and Peru are routinely extracting copper at a worldwide annual rate of 300 000 tonnes using microbes; with low-grade ores, bioleaching costs a half to a third as much as direct smelting.

Large-scale bioleaching of uranium ores is widely practised in Canada, India, the USA and the USSR. By means of bacterial leaching it is possible to recover uranium from low-grade ore (0.01–0.5% U_3O_8), which would

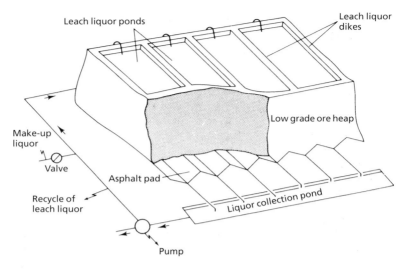

Fig. 9.8   The principle of 'mining with microbes'.

be uneconomic by any other known process. The USA alone extracts 4000 tonnes of uranium per year in this manner. Uranium is primarily used as a fuel in nuclear power generation, and microbial recovery of uranium from otherwise useless low-grade ores can be considered as an important contribution to energy production (Table 9.4). Bioleaching of uranium ores is seen to have an important contribution to the economics of nuclear power stations by providing also a means of recovery of uranium from low-grade nuclear wastes.

Continuous processes have been developed, and the control of the essential bacterial populations is easily achieved because of the acidity and limited substrate availability. Leaching technology will continue to offer more efficient and cheaper ways of extracting the increasingly scarce metals necessary for modern industry. The principal disadvantage of bioleaching is the relative slowness of the process.

Another important potential application for bacterial bioleaching is the removal of the sulphur-containing pyrite from high-sulphur coal. Little use is now made of high-sulphur coal because of the sulphur dioxide pollution that occurs with burning. However, as more and more reserves of coal are brought into use, high-sulphur coals cannot be overlooked. Thus the bacterial removal of pyrite (which contains most of the sulphur) from high-sulphur coal could well have huge economic and environmental significance.

Table 9.4. Chemical reactions associated with microbial bioleaching of low-grade uranium ores

---

Indirect oxidation of uranium ore with ferric ion catalysed by *Thiobacillus ferrooxidans*

UO_2^{2-} tetravalent uranium, insoluble oxide

$UO_2SO_4^{2-}$ hexavalent uranium (uranyl ion, UO_2^{2-}), soluble sulphate

$UO_2 + 2Fe^{3+} + SO_4^{2-} \rightarrow UO_2SO_4 + 2Fe^{2+}$

$(U^{4+} + 2Fe^{3+} \rightarrow U^{6+} + 2Fe^{2+})$

Thiobacilllus ferrooxidans re-oxidises the Fe^{2+}.

Aliphatic hydrocarbon-utilising bacteria are also being used for prospecting for petroleum deposits. Microbes will soon be commercially used to release petroleum products from oil shelf and tar sands. In all these systems there is rarely any formalised containment vessel or bioreactor. Instead, the natural geological site becomes the bioreactor, allowing water and microorganisms to flow over the ore and to be collected after natural seepage and outflow. Recycling by mechanical pumping can also be used.

Microorganisms can also be used as metal (bio) accumulators from dilute solutions. The microorgansms, bacteria, yeasts and moulds can actively uptake the metals in various ways, and such processes have a potential use in extracting rare metals from dilute solution, but it is still to be seen whether it will become an important technology.

In a similar way, microorganisms are being used to extract toxic metals from industrial effluents and reduce subsequent environmental poisoning.

Some plants have been shown to accumulate heavy metals such as nickel, cobalt, cadmium, nickel and even gold, and studies are now being carried out to assess whether such plants could be used to extract metal from soils or ores that are subeconomic for conventional mining. This area of study is called 'phytomining' and will depend on the use of hyperaccumulating plants. It is envisaged that hyperaccumulating plants would be harvested from soil containing metal, the plant material burnt to give a small volume of plant ash (bio-ore) containing high concentrations of the target metal, and the final bio-ore smelted to yield metal. Such processes are not yet commercially viable. Phytomining could well appeal to conservation movements as an alternative to opencast mining of low-grade ores.

In all these activities, multidisciplinary approaches are necessary, and new biotechnological techniques, such as designing an organism for a specific function, could yield further benefits. The overall picture of this area of biotechnology is one of rapid and exciting development. There is a growing awareness of the value of an unpolluted environment.

9.9   Environmental sustainability and clean technology

In the present chapter, attention has been drawn to the various biotechnological technologies that are being used to reduce the impact of societies' wastes on the environment. In a seminal paper, *Sustainable Biotechnology Development: From High Tech to Eco-Tech*, Moser identified how current utilisation of biotechnology is seen as a 'bolt-on' service for intrinsically unfriendly current environmental processes. While economics is the determining force for most technological changes, efforts towards enhancing environmental biotechnology must surely be viewed only as an add-on strategy.

He probingly enunciated how biotechnology with respect to environmental protection has three levels of application:

(1) *Pollution clean-up:* e.g. clean-up of oil spills and detoxification of contaminated soil; treatment of domestic and industrial waste-water supplies.
(2) *Pollution control:* e.g. recovery of heavy toxic metals from mining water; use of enzymes rather than chlorine in pulp and paper manufacture.
(3) *Pollution protection:* e.g. closed cycling practice at enzyme production plants where raw materials are renewable and waste material is a biodegradable sludge which can be used as a local fertiliser.

In past decades there has been extensive investment in the treatment of industrial waste with minimal investment in waste minimisation. The advent of the concepts of clean technology now attempts to shift attention and actions from remediation to prevention of environmental degradation. In this way it is hoped that this will lead to the emergence of technologies directed towards waste minimisation or prevention. Ideally, totally environmentally friendly technological processes would have low consumption of energy and few non-renewable raw materials (particularly fossil-fuel feedstocks) and would reduce or eliminate waste.

It is increasingly becoming evident that man's activities within the environment are far exceeding the sustainable capacity of the earth. In essence, the environmental load equals the size of the world's population × the prosperity or welfare per head of population × the environmental use per unit of prosperity (welfare). It is now apparent that in 50 years' time there will be an unavoidable requirement to reduce the environmental load 20–50 times. As it is doubtful that this can be achieved, we must either accept an increasing

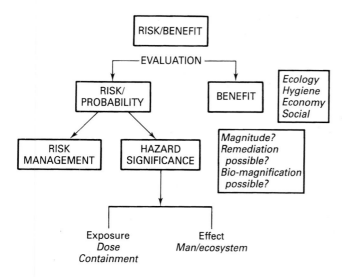

Fig. 9.9   Scheme for environmental biotechnology risk assessment (*EFB*, 1999).

erosion of environmental values and standards worldwide or set about making processes more efficient by minimising mass and energy flows. Time is running out!

All environmental biotechnology processes and products can have negative implications and such risks must be balanced against ensuring benefits. While such processes must always be put through risk assessment, it is clear that, in the light of legislative awareness and technological realism, a great amount of existing and forthcoming environmental biotechnologies should be capable of achieving maximum environmental safety (Fig. 9.9).

It is now universally accepted that environmental impact is a function of population, affluence or consumption and the technology used to create and support goods and services. If the standard of living currently achieved in the West, especially the USA, was universal, then the environmental impact would already be unsustainable.

The ecosystem must be protected from the adverse environmental effects associated with increased urbanisation and industrialisation. This will involve creative management of effluents and emissions, reducing waste generation and overall producing reliable and clean technologies where possible. Thus, there is now an increased awareness that, rather than attempt to remediate after the process, the problem should be tackled at source. Biotechnology will increasingly be seen as a means to improve many types of existing biological and chemical engineering processes which presently generate environmentally damaging by-products. There will be increased integrated bioprocess design (Chapter 4), which will develop high-quality bioprocesses that are efficient, controllable and *clean*. Biotechnology will play a central role in 'Eco-Tech' – a new technology concept 'embedding technology into the exosphere and human culture by using the whole range of biodiversity in a holistic and low-invasive way in order to achieve benefits for humankind obeying ecological principles'. (OECD, 1998).

The principal feature of future clean technologies will be to refocus attention from remediation onto prevention or minimisation of pollution and environmental degradation. Clearly, no single technology is expected to deliver clean products and processes; however, biotechnology will undoubtedly be a major driver of industrial sustainability, competing increasingly with existing chemical and physical systems in reducing material and energy consumption, and waste generation, while being economically competitive.

Sustainable development must ensure the needs of the present generation without compromising the needs of future generations.

10

Biotechnology in the agricultural and forestry industries

10.1 Introduction

Globally, agriculture and food production are challenged to produce, in a sustainable way, sufficient, healthy and safe food for the further growing world population. It is estimated that nearly eight billion people will be living on this planet by 2020, with 3.5 billion living in urban areas. To feed this world population there will need to be substantial increases in the production of the staple food commodities, namely cereals (40% increase), meat (63%) and roots and tubers (40%). At least 80% of this food will need to be produced in developing countries, yet only about 6% of new virgin soil can be brought into cultivation. Mankind must, somehow, raise yields from areas planted with cereals (two-thirds of all energy in the human diet) to approximately double the present value. Consequently, there can be no alternative other than to plan, with modern scientific inputs, new agricultural systems that are sustainable yet intensive. Whereas in the last great 'green revolution' in agriculture in the 1960s to 1970s, the environment was adapted to the plant by increased use of fertilisers, biocides, irrigation, etc., modern sustainable agriculture must increasingly adapt the plant to the environment, breeding high-yielding crops that can grow in places deficient in nitrogen or water, and where plant diseases and pests prevail. Many aspects of modern biotechnology are, and will increasingly be, applied to agriculture.

Agriculture continues to be the world's largest single industry and, in advanced societies like the USA, agriculture contributes over 20% of total gross national production. In developed economies agriculture relies heavily on technology to achieve productivity and profitability. Agriculture in many parts of the world is undergoing a major strategic restructuring to achieve vertical integration between production and ultimate utilisation. Whereas the food processor would formerly buy raw agricultural products on the commodity market, they are increasingly establishing breeding programmes to create the desired raw materials with the specific traits required for higher value processing. Genetic engineering is creating a revolution in agriculture, allowing an ever-increasing range of plants and animals. There will be increased stability in the marketplace and much less wastage. Agricultural biotechnology will allow higher quality standards with lower costs of production.

Agriculture is a politically sensitive area with many selective trade barriers and protectionist policies. In many parts of the world, e.g. Europe and the USA, agriculture is a highly efficient industry and continues to demonstrate annual increases in productivity. In contrast, many countries are still not self-sufficient in food production owing to many reasons, such as lack of good agricultural practices, hostile or changing climate, or political instability. Many countries are intrinsically poor and lack the ability to take advantage of new agricultural practices and biotechnology. This can only be remedied when the advanced nations make available the training programmes and financial investments required. However, much is already taking place through agencies such as the World Bank and the EU.

10.2　Plant biotechnology

Plants are the primary source of food for the human race and only by correct management of plant agriculture can the present human populations continue to be fed. Surprisingly, only a relatively few plant species have been brought into agricultural practice. While there are at least 300 000 known plant species, only a few hundred have had any significant impact on agriculture. Manipulating the genetic constitution of plants and then selecting the characteristics that are best suited to human needs has prevailed throughout the history of agriculture. The flow of energy from sunlight through plant photosynthesis is at the heart of the importance of plants in the world economy. In the highly technology-driven world that we now live in, the links between plants and people are easily overlooked (Fig. 10.1).

Since early times, man has sought to improve the quality and productivity of agriculturally important plants. This was done by selection and traditional breeding procedures – a painstakingly slow and difficult process. But it has been a remarkably successful commitment, as witnessed by the high quality of the present food plants, such as corn, rice, wheat, and potato – all far removed

INPUTS

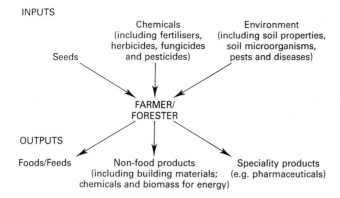

Fig. 10.1   A scheme illustrating the production and uses of plants (adapted from Organisation for Economic Cooperation and Development, 1992).

from their ancestral beginnings. Traditional breeding programmes involving natural or induced mutations and sexual crosses will continue to dominate the approach to improve the agronomic characteristics of food crops but will be increasingly augmented by new techniques incorporating micropropagation, protoplast fusion and genetic engineering.

The rate of genetic improvement has been historically restricted by the number of suitable genes available and the ability to form and propagate the improved strains. However, by the nature of modern genomics, more useful genes from plants and other sources are now becoming available, together with the development of methods for transforming and then expressing those genes in appropriate crop strains. A major challenge will be to try to understand how to control the way genes act in concert to produce crop traits of value to farmers, processors and consumers.

As early as 1939 it became possible to isolate small numbers of cells from certain plants and to keep them alive indefinitely in artificial cultivation. The cultivation of these tissues required the presence of a plant hormone which allowed the cells to propagate in an unorganised manner, resulting in an amorphous mass of cells. Advances were soon made in cultivation techniques, achieving rapid growth rates in chemically defined media. These individuals or groups of cells were treated like microbial suspensions and were able to grow under aerated and shaken conditions, initially in flasks but subsequently in large traditional bioreactors. (By this method it is possible to produce important secondary metabolites with high commercial value; Table 10.1.)

The next major advance in plant cell culture was to achieve the complete reversal of this process by causing these individual plant cells to go through

Table 10.1. Potential markets for plant secondary products

Compound	Use	Estimated retail market ($ million)
Vinblastine/vincristine	Leukaemia	18–20 (US)
Ajmalicine	Circulatory problems	5–25 (world)
Digitalis	Heart disorders	20–55 (US)
Quinine	Malaria; flavour	5–10 (US)
Codeine	Sedative	50 (US)
Jasmine	Fragrance	0.5 (world)
Pyrethrins	Insecticide	20 (world)
Spearmint	Flavour; fragrance	85–90 (world)

a developmental programme from individual plant cells to tissues, to organs, and finally to entire plants. In this way it has become possible to clone plant cells.

Rapid, large-scale clonal propagation of many plant species, including trees, is now feasible. Small tissue explants of many species can be aseptically removed from the parent plant and artificially maintained and increased in number by suitable control of the medium. The process can be rapid and produces high-quality, uniform plants. Outstanding examples of this technology have been the recent successful cloning of oil palms and coffee plants from callus tissues, producing unlimited numbers of stable types. This area of micropropagation not only allows rapid propagation or mass production of identical clones of plant species but also has the following uses:

(1) elimination of viruses and other pathogens;
(2) storage of essential germ plasm instead of conventional seeds;
(3) embryo rescue;
(4) production of haploids by anther and ovary culture (gametoclonal variants), useful for cereals.

It is now possible to take plant cells and subject them to the battery of manipulative techniques long practised in industrial microbiology, e.g. mutation, strain selection and process development. Thus the genetic diversity of plants may be altered, without the normal sexual process of fertilisation, by production of haploid, triploid and tetraploid cells, by the use of protoplast fusion between different species and even genera, and by transformation, i.e. transferring DNA from one plant cell (or even another type of organism) into

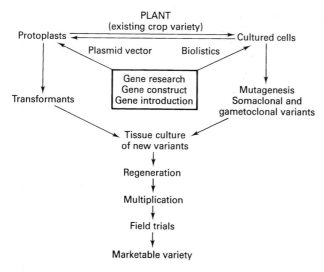

Fig. 10.2 Experimental approaches used to create new plant varieties by biotechnology.

the cells of another. The techniques of recombinant DNA technology are now practically available to the plant technologist (Fig. 10.2).

Protoplasts can be produced from most plant cells by digesting away the cell wall and maintaining the protoplasts in a suitable osmotic medium. Many types of protoplasts can be induced to re-form cell walls and to divide to form cell colonies. Some plants, including potato, pepper, tobacco and tomato, can be fully regenerated from protoplasts. Full regeneration for important cereal crops is not yet possible. Some protoplasts may be fused with other species, allowing a novel mixing of genetic traits.

With tissue culture of callus or large structures, regeneration mainly leads to uniformity of plants. In contrast, regeneration from single plant cells or protoplasts can often be accompanied by minor or extensive changes in the final plant phenotype. This has been termed '*somoclonal variation*' and is widely used as a means of crop improvement, in particular with respect to yield and disease resistance (Fig. 10.2).

The first practical system for genetically manipulating plants occurred in 1983 with the ability of the bacterium *Agrobacterium tumifaciens* to transfer part of its Ti plasmid (T-DNA) into the host plant genome (DNA). In this way foreign genes can be inserted into the plasmid DNA and then integrated into the plant genome. Transformants can be identified by selection methods, adult plants reconstituted from the transfected cells, and the new genetic

Table 10.2. Crops into which single purified genes have been introduced

Cereals	Beverage plants	Fibre	Legumes/ oil seeds	Vegetables, fruits	Flowers	Pasture	Trees
Rice	Coffee	Cotton	Linseed	Carrot	Rose	Lucerne	White spruce
Maize		Flax	Soya bean	Tomato	Chrysanthemum	Orchid Grass	Walnut
Wheat			Rape	Strawberry	Carnation		Apple
Rye			Sunflower	Celery	Geranium		
			Canola	Cauliflower			
			Palm	Tobacco			
				Sugar beet			
				Cucumber			
				Potato			

Note: this list is constantly being extended.
Adapted from Organisation for Economic Cooperation and Development (1992).

material transmitted as a Mendelian trait. Nowadays, the Ti plasmid-derived vector is used routinely in laboratories throughout the world for transforming dicotyledon crop plants. This method was unsuitable for most monocotyledon crop plants such as maize, wheat and rice. Successful gene transfer into the monocotyledon crop plants was achieved by biolistics or 'particle gun', which was used to bombard plant cells with DNA (genes) – coated particles. In this way the microprojectiles penetrated the cell walls and delivered the DNA into the nucleus. The intact cells could be regenerated into whole plants (Fig. 10.2).

By these methods it is now possible to introduce advantageous new traits into almost any plant species, and a wide range of agricultural crop plants have been manipulated (Table 10.2).

Ti plasmids have also been used to insert 'antisense genes' in order to negate the functions of specific plant genes concerned with an undesirable phenotype. Such genes are produced by reversing the orientation of a gene in relationship to its promoter. The transcribed product cannot be translated into a normal protein, thus inhibiting that function within the plant.

What are the current main goals for the application of genetic engineering to plant agriculture? In essence, genetic engineering releases the plant breeder from two major constraints:

(1) limits imposed by interspecific barriers, and
(2) lack of precision inherent in traditional breeding methods.

Presently, genetic engineering methods allow the introduction of single-gene characteristics into plant cells, and this later should extend to multiple genes and, indeed, whole biochemical pathways. The main introduced improvements will initially include:

(1) improved resistance to specific herbicides;
(2) improved resistance to insect pests and microbial diseases;
(3) improved post-harvest characteristics.

Improved resistance to specific herbicides

The killing of plant weed species by the application of selective herbicides gives a growth advantage to commercial crop plants. Such compounds have been designed to disrupt the growth of certain weed species without affecting the particular crop plant. The annual global herbicide market is approximately $6 billion. However, there is increasing opposition to the continued use of such chemical compounds from environmental and human health considerations. Herbicide-tolerant crop plants have now been produced by genetically engineering genes that are resistant to specific herbicides. This has been viewed as a way of producing more effective, less costly and more environmentally compatible weed control. This will permit reduced overall herbicide use, and a return to broad-spectrum herbicides which have a low mammalian toxicity and which are rapidly degraded by soil microorganisms. Successful crops so far in use include the potato and oil-seed rape. Weed control is an indispensable aspect of modern agriculture.

Improved resistance to insect pests and microbial diseases

Gene transfer into crop plants to impart insect or microbial resistance is a major new area of research towards plant protection. Most efforts have been directed towards protecting standing crops in the field while little attention has yet been given to insect pests in post-harvest storage, where huge losses can occur, particularly in developing countries. Genes (Bt) from *Bacillus thuringiensis* have been introduced into several crops, including tomato and cotton, and field testing has demonstrated impressive results against many pests.

Microbial diseases, in particular fungal and viral diseases, remain one of the major factors limiting crop productivity worldwide, with continuing huge losses set against large cash inputs for pesticide treatment. Global estimates of losses due to plant diseases in 1987 were approximately US$90 billion. Much improved resistance to viruses by the integration of genes for viral coat proteins has now been achieved in several crop plants, particularly rice. These approaches could well be the most advantageous aspects of all plant biotechnology. The necessary widespread use of insecticides, fungicides and pesticides for crop protection undoubtedly has damaging effects on the environment and consequently it is imperative to improve the control of pests and diseases by genetic and other rational alternative means.

Improved post-harvest characteristics

Losses during storage and transport of some crops can be as high as 40% in the USA and Europe and as high as 80% elsewhere. While a great deal of this loss will be due to diseases and pests with soft fruits and vegetables, there can be bruising, heat and cold damage, over-ripeness, off flavours and odours, etc. Most of these physiological changes result from endogenous enzyme activity. Can such activity be genetically stopped or slowed down? In the tomato, the enzyme polygalacturonase breaks down cell wall constituents, leading to softening of the fruit during ripening. This process is independent of colour development. In normal conditions, if the tomato is left to ripen on the vine and develop full colour, the softening process is also occurring, thus creating an easily bruised and damaged fruit on shipment. By inhibiting the polygalacturonase enzyme by antisense genes, the tomato can remain on the vine until mature and be transported in a firm solid state. The Flavo Savr tomato has been engineered by Calgene in the USA with improved flavour and keepability and is now marketed in the USA. The current US market for fresh tomatoes is US$3.5 billion. Such principles will now be used in a wide variety of soft fruits. Other studies are considering ethylene synthesis/inhibition as a means of controlling fruit and flavour maturation.

Genetic manipulation of flower and leaf colour, abundance of flowers, perfume and shape are now major targets for the decorative plant industries. In the Netherlands there is an annual market in cut flowers in excess of $1.5 billion.

Production of high-value oil products

There is increased interest in the genetic modification of oil-producing plants such as soya bean, rape and canola in order to produce a wide range of industrial lubricants, cosmetic compounds, biodegradable detergents, etc.

Table 10.3. Approximate annual world production of some plant-derived agricultural products

Sector	Product	Tonnes
Food and feed	Cereals	1.8 billion
	Sugar	120 million
	Crude starch	1.0 billion
Materials	Harvested wood	1.6 billion
	Paper	200 million
	Cotton	16 million
Chemical	Plant oils	43 million
	Natural rubber	4 million
Others	Tobacco	4 million

Adapted from Organisation for Economic Cooperation and Development (1992).

The proportion of plant agricultural production directed towards non-food uses has now passed 20% in many developed countries, e.g. cotton, tobacco, natural rubber and, of course, wood. The discovery that plants can synthesise functional human antibody fragments opens up a whole new area for plant biotechnology. The use of plants as antibody factories will avoid the often controversial industrial sacrificial use of animals but also the possible transfer of viruses and prions.

The first stages of the plant biotechnology revolution have now arrived and are being assessed by a somewhat sceptical and unprepared public. Successful commercial products will need to meet a genuine market need. The approximate annual world production of some agricultural products is shown in Table 10.3.

The correlation and coordination of the vast quantities of information molecular researchers are generating will involve a substantial effort in bioinformatics. This will be essential to link all operations in crop development on the molecular constitution of plants and on the interactions between molecules. While genomics has dominated plant research in the last two decades, plant proteomics has now come of age.

As will be discussed later, there has been much unjust opposition to plant genetic engineering by a vocal minority, especially in Europe. To argue that this new technology is not required in the food-affluent western countries does great disservice to the vast majority of people in the developing world. Sustainable agriculture will not be possible in many developing countries

Table 10.4. Traits of transgenic plants that would find uses in developing countries

Insect resistance
Virus resistance
Beta-carotene enrichment (to correct vitamin A deficiency and infantile blindness)
Nutritional enrichment in oil or starch or essential amino acids
Tailored fatty acid profiles (oil crops)
Animal feeds containing cellulases, phospholipases and toxin-degrading enzymes (more digestibility)
Antigen producing (edible oral vaccines)
Ripening delayed (for melons, etc., to prevent rotting and storage problems)
Resistance to bacterial and fungal diseases
Resistance to water stress
Salt tolerance
Aluminium and manganese tolerance (for use in acidic soils)

From Salamini (1999).

without the use *and* availability of creative plant genetic engineering. There is not a choice – it is obligatory. The constrictions now envisaged by these 'full-stomach' sceptics will damage the full development of this scientific area and will, undoubtedly, in the near future, lead to unprecedented sufferings. Some of the valuable traits that would benefit developing countries are listed in Table 10.4.

10.3   Forest biotechnology

Throughout the world there is an escalation in demand for wood-derived products and many major countries such as Europe, India and Japan are now in deficit. This will be further compounded by increased pollution such as 'acid rain' and the huge losses now occurring in the rainforests of South America and Asia by indiscriminate felling. Worldwide forests are diminishing while the demand for their products, such as pulp and paper industries, construction, fuel and other requirements, is increasing. Forest trees have not had the research and management that cultivated crops, such as coffee, citrus, rubber, coconut and others, have received, and are more often viewed as self-regenerating resources that need little cultivation. This is in sharp contrast to most other plant crops which have been tailored to accommodate human needs through extensive breeding programmes. Furthermore, resulting from their long generation times, there is a paucity of information on tree genetics, and modern plant-breeding strategies may not be truly relevant.

However, biotechnology will play an important role in achieving an increase in production as well as in bringing major improvements to the quality of the trees. Tissue-culture technology, such as micropropagation, somatic embryo-genesis (induction of single cells or cell aggregates to develop into embryo-like structures from which a shoot and root develop), selection of somoclonal and gametoclonal variants, and gene transfer, are being developed to improve forests (Fig. 10.2). Trees have long generation times and, as a consequence, genetic improvements will be slow. Loblolly pine has been transformed by *Agrobacterium tumefaciens* and this may allow gene transfer techniques that are similar to those used with other plant species.

Targets for tree improvement are well recognised, namely: apical domi-nance; wood quality; disease, pest and herbicide resistance; and nutrient use. While herbicide- and insect-resistant crops are becoming available, the genes involved have yet to be characterised. Future focus will involve functional gen-omics applying microarray technology to define differentially expressed genes.

Increased yields is the prime target of all forestry sectors, with emphasis on shorter cycle times. It is well recognised that tree productivity correlates with solar input and temperature; thus a forest the size of Sweden in Brazil would satisfy current global wood needs. If high-yielding forests can be achieved by selective breeding programmes, it could lead to a doubling of present-day plantation productivity (estimated at 1.5 million cubic metres per year) while halving the land area required. If commercial wood production could be confined to smaller landbase and achieve a sustainable system, natural forests could then be left for biological diversity and public amenity. Table 10.5 identifies some potential impacts of biotechnology on forestry.

10.4   Biological control

The use of chemical pesticides has led to dramatic improvements in the pro-duction levels of agriculture and forestry. Their widespread use is the dominant reason that fewer people can now produce more food at less cost than ever previously. The pesticide market is dominated by synthetic chemicals and will undoubtedly remain so. However, consumers are becoming increasingly con-cerned about food quality and possible carry-over of pesticide residues into food products. Biotechnologists are now actively examining alternatives to chemical pesticides as a means of controlling agricultural pests and diseases. An obvious approach would be to use naturally occurring biological means of controlling these problems. It is a fact of life that all organisms have their own specific diseases and predators. In the present context, biological control will refer to the use of microorganisms applied in the field to control pests

Table 10.5. The potential impact of biotechnology on forestry

Industry demands	Enhanced growth rate and decreases in rotation time Feedstock suited to harvesting and handling capacity (straight trunks, short limbs) Uniformity of feed stocks
Biological/biotechnological challenges	Tree genomes are larger Long generation times Some desirable traits genetically complex Uniformity already achievable by cloned forestry Price of feedstock critical
Product/technology benefits	Increased yield Shorter generation times Pest resistance Enhanced cold-, drought-resistance
Deliverable by 2020	Correlation of genetic markers and desirable traits Methods for mass propagation of superior germ plasm Environmentally acceptable systems for testing and deployment of genetically modified trees Environmentally acceptable systems for testing and deployment of genetically modified trees

From Robinson (1999).

and diseases. In a similar way, insect predators can also be used for control purposes.

Biological pest control has not proved to be as effective or economical as chemical control. Problems associated with the use of biocontrol to manage pest problems include: slow, delayed and/or inadequate activity; a restricted pest-control spectrum; inconsistent activity across different environments; and high costs involved in production and rearing of biological control agents (BCAs).

The most successful BCA is *Bacillus thuringiensis*, a spore-forming bacterium containing crystalline protein inclusions. The proteins are highly toxic to insect pests but specific in their activity. They have been widely used for over 30 years against *Lepidoptera* (caterpillar) pests. The commercial application of these biopesticides is usually as formulations of spores and crystalline inclusions of disrupted *B. thuringiensis* and are applied at 10–15 g/acre or about 10^{20} molecules/acre.

In recent years the toxin genes have been isolated and sequenced and recombinant DNA-based products produced and approved. These genes have also been incorporated into various plant species and expressed in the plant tissue. This now offers the farmer either direct application of the microbial biopesticides or protection of the plant directly by toxic gene expression in the plant tissue. A large number of companies are now involved in the research, development and production of *B. thuringiensis* toxins. In most cases the companies are relatively small, innovative and research-driven, but tend to form associations with well-established agrochemical companies. While the *B. thuringiensis* (Bt) toxins dominate the market, there are many examples of viral and fungal biopesticides that are achieving an increased market share.

Sadly, evidence has now accumulated that insect resistance to Bt toxin has developed from the transgenic plants, whereas there was no resistance developed from the direct application of the toxin. According to entomologists, Bt insect-resistance management plans should include 'refuges' or fields of non-Bt plants where populations of insects will not encounter the toxin and will, therefore, fail to develop resistance to it. If the refuges are suitably sized and sufficiently close to the fields of transgenic plants, any resistant insects will be likely to breed with non-resistant insects, diluting the trait out of the pest population. Refuge size should be 10–50% of the total crop, depending on the plant, region and whether or not pesticides were used on the refuge.

In recent years the concept of integrated pest management (IPM) has evolved and is a multidisciplinary, ecological approach to the management of pest populations which makes use of a variety of control tactics compatible in a single-pest management system. Consequently, IPM is not dependent on any one control tactic or procedure. Currently, insecticides remain a primary agricultural pest-control approach and present IPM methods involve the use of pesticides, together with various BCAs and procedures.

Biological control relies on the use of selected natural predators from the native range of a given pest to reduce the pest's negative effects. Such natural enemies of the targeted pest species can include pathogenic viruses, bacteria and fungi, together with protozoal parasites. The potential use of biotechnology in an IPM system is considerable. A widely used approach has been to modify pest arthropods by radiation and chemosterilisation, induction of various chromosomal aberrations, hybrid sterility and genetic incompatibility.

Table 10.6. Requirements for a microorganism to be a successful biological control agent (BCA)

(1) It must have a substantial market-size and consumer demand.
(2) It must be equal to, or better than, chemical pesticides in performance and persistence.
(3) The product must be safe, with low mammalian toxicity and little effect on non-target species.
(4) It should remain stable on storage.
(5) Mass production by bioprocess technology should be cheap.
(6) BCAs should be applied using conventional technology without recourse to major changes in current agricultural practices.

Genetic engineering does not yet appear to be involved in biological control. What is urgently required is a broad-host-range insect transformation system that could provide the necessary tools to create insect modifications. Some foreign gene transfer has been achieved for some insects, including medflies, silkworms, honeybees and mosquitoes. Such ultimate use of genetically modified organisms for biological control requires their eventual release into the environment, and this would be classified as 'deliberate release'.

The commercial potential for these products will be determined by their efficacy and cost–benefit ratios when compared with synthetic chemicals, ease of use and spectrum of activity (Table 10.6). The comparisons between chemical and microbial pesticides are shown in Table 10.7.

It is anticipated that BCAs may ultimately increase their market share of global pesticide applications to about 5%. However, should consumer opinion move strongly against chemical pesticides then the BCA option will emerge as a meaningful alternative.

10.5　Animal biotechnology

Animal agriculture in the form of cattle, pigs, sheep, poultry and fish represents a major aspect of food production worldwide. While many of these animals are produced for their meat alone, others contribute to human nutrition by way of milk and egg production. In the developed world animal production is highly intensified and technologically driven. Animal production will reflect on quality of feed, availability and need of growth hormones, pesticides, antibiotics

Table 10.7. Chemical versus microbial pesticides

	Chemical pesticide	Microbial pesticide
Product use		
Speed of action	Usually rapid	Can be slow
Killing efficacy	Often 100%	Usually 90–95%
Spectrum of effect	Generally broad	Generally narrow
Resistance of target organism	Often developed	Not yet seen
Product safety		
Toxicological testing	Lengthy and costly	Low cost
Environmental hazards	Many well-known examples	None yet shown
Residues	Interval to harvest usually required	Crop may be harvested immediately

and vaccines, good animal husbandry and welfare, and increasingly selective breeding, molecular biology, embryo manipulation and gene transfer.

As with plant agriculture, early animal breeders sought to identify worthwhile properties in animals and to perpetuate them into future offspring. Selective breeding aims to increase the frequency of a large number of genes that work together with the remainder of the animal's genes or genome to produce the desired phenotype. For example, between 1945 and 1993, selective breeding increased milk production of the average dairy cow by a factor of 3. Further, when we consider the huge variety of dogs, it should be remembered that they are all one species, capable of easily interbreeding, and that the present varieties have arisen by carefully controlled selective breeding programmes. For many farm animals, conventional breeding has already achieved high-producing animals, but it is increasingly apparent that the increases in productivity possible by this means would now appear to be approaching a plateau. To sustain an ever-increasing world population, ways must be achieved to meet this increasing demand for animal products.

Genetic engineering for transgenic animals

Selective breeding is a painfully slow process and, especially with larger animals with long gestation periods, can take many years to establish desired phenotypic changes. However, the advent of recombinant DNA technology

Table 10.8. Anticipated changes involving transgenic animals

Efficiency of meat production
Improved quality of meat
Milk quality and quantity
Egg production
Wool quality and quantity
Disease resistance in animals
Production of low-cost pharmaceuticals and biologicals

and its application to animal breeding programmes could greatly increase the speed and range of selective breeding. The first recorded example of the transfer of a foreign gene into an animal by recombinant DNA technology was the insertion and expression of a rat gene for growth hormone into a mouse. The subsequent progeny were all much larger than the parents. This 'Super Mouse' gained much public attention as it was the first example of a transgenic animal, i.e. animals that have acquired novel genetic material by artificial means rather than by the normal route of sexual reproduction.

Subsequently, there has been extensive speculation on the economic potential of transgenic farm animals and there can be little doubt that this should become a highly lucrative worldwide industry with great benefits to mankind. However, as will be discussed in Chapter 14, it is perhaps the most controversial of all areas of modern biotechnology. Notwithstanding, some of the main opportunities where this new technology can be envisaged with animal breeding programmes are listed in Table 10.8. Of particular relevance will be improvements in meat production from a wide range of farmed animals, including fish, improved milk yields and quality, and disease-free animals. Undoubtedly, the most unusual but commercially feasible projects are the use of certain lactating animals such as sheep, pigs, rabbits and cows to produce novel secretions of human proteins in their milk which can then be extracted and used pharmaceutically.

How can novel DNA be incorporated into animal genomes and then stably inherited into the offspring? At the present time the most successful method for gene transfer into livestock is by microinjection into the pronucleus of fertilised eggs. Microinjection techniques make use of finely constructed glass needles which allow the injection of purified DNA into the fertilised eggs of the chosen species. The eggs are then surgically transferred into hormonally synchronised surrogate mothers (Table 10.9). Unlike mice and pigs,

Table 10.9. Steps necessary to establish transgenic animals

- Identification and construction of foreign gene (genetic engineering)
- Microinjection of DNA directly into the pronucleus of a single fertilised egg
- Implantation of these engineered cells into surrogate mothers
- Bringing the developing embryo to term
- Proving that the foreign DNA has been stably and heritably incorporated into the DNA of at least some of the newborn offspring
- Demonstrating that the gene is sufficiently regulated so as to function in its new environment

litter size is limited to one or two in sheep and cattle and, therefore, large numbers of animals have to be employed as recipients of the microinjected eggs.

Transgenic pigs, sheep and cattle have now been obtained, although the frequency of success is only about 1% compared with 2–5% with mice. This low efficiency of the technology will continue to exert some limitation to wider acceptance. However, with fish, the eggs are fertilised externally and this eliminates many of the complicated techniques required in mammals to harvest ova, fertilise them, and then introduce the embryos into foster mothers. Successful fish transgenics can be as high as 70%.

The ultimate goal of animal breeders will be to introduce specific economically important traits into commercial livestock (Table 10.8). However, the knowledge of the mechanisms regulating gene expression in higher animals is limited and this restricts the ability to construct transgenic animals.

A novel and commercially realistic use of transgenic animals will be the production of human proteins/pharmaceuticals in transgenic lactating animals. Transgenic constructs that allow the mammary glands of lactating animals to secrete high-value human proteins are now possible and will undoubtedly be the first truly commercial use of transgenic animals for product formation. The animals will in fact become bioreactors, producing pharmaceutical products previously only produced in culture by transgenic microorganisms. Gene constructs for human factors IX or α-1 antitrypsin (some haemophiliacs lack a blood-clotting agent called 'factor IX') have been successfully inserted into the sheep genome and, while expression levels are still low, factor IX is present and the trait is heritable. The potential of transgenic animals to secrete a wide range of commercially valuable healthcare products is almost unlimited and should be realised in the future. Pharmaceutically used transgenic sheep will not be allowed to enter the human food chain, thus removing possible public outcry concerning the consumption (cannibalism) of the human gene inserts

(Chapter 14). Contrary to some popular viewpoints, transgenic animal studies are not about producing animal monsters and freaks but, rather, about introducing specific, economically significant traits into livestock which will have benefits to mankind. Transgenic animals have also contributed hugely to the understanding of gene function in animal species.

In the 1950s, scientists removed the nuclei from frogs' eggs, replaced them with somatic nuclei from embryos, and succeeded in raising adult frogs. This was then followed by serial transplantations using the nuclei from the transplanted embryos for more transplantations. Consequently, all the embryos could be considered to have identical nuclei; this was termed '*nuclear cloning*'. In the 1990s, Dolly the sheep was created in Scotland from a nucleus derived from an adult ewe inserted into an enucleated oocyte. This subsequently led to huge public interest and debate, fuelled by exaggerated media coverage, on the possible 'cloning' of human beings. The debate continues. Sadly, Dolly the sheep recently died somewhat earlier than expected and, while the cause of death may well have been due to natural causes, it must also be determined whether the original nucleus from the donor ewe already carried an age factor, thus reducing the normal lifespan of the sheep.

While the term 'clone' has been used for these mammals and frogs, it should be correctly termed '*somatic cell nuclear transfer*'. It should be noted that animals derived in this way will also contain mitochondrial genes from the egg. Undoubtedly, the most significant results of the 'Dolly study' were that an adult mammalian cell can reactivate dormant genetic instructions that have been shut down as it divides, specialises and ages, and can then become a new life force.

Genetically engineered hormones and vaccines

The pituitary gland of animals secretes growth hormones which can have major influence on how the animal grows and, in lactating animals, on milk production. In the 1980s the gene responsible for bovine growth hormone (somatotropin) production (BST) was successfully isolated and transferred into bacterial cells to produce large quantities of BST. When cows were injected with about 30 mg BST there was significant increase in milk production (10–30%), but continued increased yields depended on regular injections. Such improvements in milk production could lead to fewer animals producing the same volume of milk. There is no evidence of increased concentrations of BST in the milk, nor that the constituents of milk are in any way altered. Comparable studies with genetically engineered pig somatotropin (PST) have shown that body fat can be reduced by up to 80% and feed efficiency increased by

20%. The approval of BST by the Food and Drug Administration in November, 1993, represented the first biotechnology-derived pharmaceutical to be commercialised for animal agriculture in the USA.

BST is the first genetically engineered product in agriculture which has been intensively examined for its economic impact. This is due mainly to the vast importance of milk to most western economies and the positive product image of milk for human health. Animal welfare is also of major current concern.

From a scientific point of view, BST has been clearly demonstrated to be a safe product and is now permitted in many countries, in particular the USA, where it is marketed by Monsanto under the tradename '*Posilac*'. Many consumer organisations continue to oppose the use of this method. In Europe, the European commissioners have recommended a continuation of the earlier ban for a further 5 years for reasons which are more politically based than for health and safety reasons. In Europe, struggling to control over-production of milk, is a milk-boosting hormone really needed? Furthermore, the large numbers of small dairy farmers who might go out of business have considerable political impact.

From an animal welfare consideration there is now evidence that pigs transgenic for PST suffered skeletal and joint problems, while cows have increased mastitis. Some would consider that BST and PST were the wrong biotechnology-derived products to lead the way for public acceptance of new biotechnology. The public viewpoint of this biotechnology product is that it has been profit-driven and not need-driven. Much has been learned from this product which may be applicable to the introduction of other new biotechnology products in agriculture.

Animal vaccine production has been developed against many microbial diseases and uses methods previously described in Chapter 8. Animal diseases represent a major cause of suffering in all forms of animal farming and, if disease could be reduced or eliminated, then animal welfare as well as yields would improve. By improving the health of the animals (e.g. in intensive farming) the number of animals required to give the same final yield could be reduced.

The production of genetically engineered animal vaccines has been a major, if somewhat unheralded, success story in biotechnology. Numerous vaccines have been developed for specific cattle, pig, poultry, sheep and fish diseases. The commercial success is considerable, though not dramatic, but has led to much reduction in animal hardship. A new genetically engineered vaccine against rabies is now being scattered in chicken heads in many parts of Europe where rabies is endemic in the wildlife. The future for this type of disease prevention is immense.

Animal organs for human patients

In the last few decades medical skills have permitted a wide range of human organ transplants, such as kidneys, hearts, lungs and livers. However, throughout the world there are massive waiting lists with donors falling far short of demand. Can suitable animal organs be a serious option? Two international companies, together with many research institutions, have been striving to meet the demand by tailoring pigs so that their organs could save human lives. Analysts believe the market could be worth £5 billion for solid organs alone, with at least the same again possible from cellular therapies, e.g. transplantable cells that could produce insulin for the treatment of diabetes.

Previous attempts at transplanting animal organs into humans have been unsuccessful owing to rejection by the human immune system. The human immune system recognises that the animal organ is 'foreign' and sets in motion a 'hyperacute' rejection. An important reason for this rejection can be related to an enzyme present in all animals but not in man – α-1,3 galactosyl transferase – which adds a sugar to the surface of all animal (pig) cells. It is this sugar that is recognised by the human immune system and causes rapid allergic response.

The recent renewed interest in the potential use of animal organs for transplants relates to the birth of piglets in which the transferase enzyme has been deleted from their genome. Enzyme deletion can only be achieved in single cells and the piglets have been produced by cloning from these single cells, just as Dolly the sheep was created. These ongoing studies are an essential step forward but not the final solution. It is believed that at least three more genes will need to be deleted to deal with all stages of rejection.

Apart from rejection, scientists will have to be concerned about infection, since pigs carry viruses that could potentially cause human disease or epidemics. However, pig cells have already been used in various experiments with humans, with no signs of porcine retroviruses. Much still needs to be done, but this is undoubtedly a major step forward for animal/human transplants. Ethical considerations will also be a source of much debate.

10.6   Diagnostics in agriculture

In traditional analytical methods applied to plant and animal agriculture, be it chemical or microbiological, the primary aim has been to isolate or separate out the analyte from the complex chemical milieu of the sample. Such methods

Table 10.10. Criteria required for successful rapid methods of agricultural analysis

- Fast, accurate and reliable
- Simple to operate and have low running costs
- Readily available and stable reagents
- Minimal labour requirements
- High degree of sensitivity and specificity

normally require an operator of considerable chemical analytical experience, and are time consuming and expensive. However, new methods based on biotechnologically derived techniques are revolutionising many aspects of agricultural analysis, not only by being able to equal the sensitivity of the established methods but also by being able to carry out many determinations *in situ* without the need for complex isolation procedures. Furthermore, these methods are usually cheaper, more easily adapted to automation and more rapid. Often, too, they can be performed by relatively unskilled operators (Table 10.10).

In the present context, the impact of three new biotechnologically derived rapid methods – namely, immunoassays, DNA probes and biosensors – will be examined in the context of plant and veterinary diseases and the physiological monitoring of animals. In almost all cases these new rapid methods were first developed with the massive human healthcare market in mind, where economic rewards were obvious, with huge sales anticipated in hospitals and surgeries and for home care and monitoring (Chapter 8). The veterinary market has also been a highly profitable activity, while in plant agriculture the new methods are increasingly being used.

Immunoassays in general, but specifically those using monoclonal antibodies, are widely recognised for their commercial success in clinical and veterinary diagnostics. Indeed, these diagnostic tests make up a major part of new biotechnological products presently on the market. Immunoassays differ from other analytical methods in that the high technology resides in the molecules rather than in the apparatus. Nucleic acid probe technology is based on the principle of hybridisation of complementary sequences of DNA or of DNA and RNA. The respective nucleotide strands must have exact, corresponding sequences of nucleotide bases for exact hybridisation or alignment to occur; thus a given strand can hybridise only with its complementary strand. This high level of specificity has now been directed at identifying microorganisms in complex mixtures – the DNA probe or hybridisation assay.

Table 10.11. Successful and anticipated uses of rapid diagnostic methods with animal diseases

Animal type	Rapid diagnostic methods used for:
Companion animals	Feline leukaemia, canine heartworm, rheumatoid arthritis
Poultry	Screening of avian retrovirus; coccidiosis, salmonellosis, respiratory infections
Large animals	Trichinosis, mastitis, leukaemia, brucellosis, rinderpest, trypanosomiasis, swine fever, foot-and-mouth virus

Using these diagnostic methods it is now possible to detect microbial diseases in animals at very low levels of infection in body fluids or tissues and to be able to isolate such animals before they become infectious. A wide range of animal diseases can now be more easily monitored by 'user friendly' diagnostic kits applied by the veterinarian or the farmer. Early diagnosis can be an essential prerequisite for containment and elimination of infectious diseases (Table 10.11).

One of the largest areas of application for diagnostic kits is in measuring fertility hormones in animal blood or milk, e.g. progesterone, oestrogen sulphate or equine gonadotrophin. Illegal use of growth hormones and antibiotics can also be monitored. Several hundred different diagnostic kits are now available worldwide.

Immunochemical technology using monoclonal antibodies is now widely used for the analysis of pesticide residues in foods, together with toxic microbial products such as mycotoxins. Specific plant diseases can now be detected in a crop at very early stages and appropriate treatment applied earlier. Such methods can also be used to analyse the phytosanitary quality of seed products for sale and to certify that potatoes, bulbs, fruit trees and ornamental plants are disease-free. These methods now allow more efficient crop breeding and international trade. Genetic fingerprinting now allows easy differentiation between plant varieties.

Several pre- and post-harvest problems are of major concern in food production, distribution, processing and subsequent storage and handling. It has been estimated that, globally, 30–60% of total food produced is lost during this process. The main problems include pests and diseases, senescence in fruits and vegetables, chemical and biochemical degradation of fruits, vegetables, dairy and meat products, and microbial spoilage. Rapid screening tests are now increasingly used to monitor food from field to table for quality and safety. Rapid diagnostic methods must also be advantageous in the event of any possible chemical or microbiological contamination of crops and the general food supply by bioterrorism.

The cost of microbial diseases on world plant production is estimated at £50 billion annually. However, present estimates consider that only a relatively small part of this would be suitable for the use of immunodiagnostics. It is now not difficult to develop antibodies specific to known fungal, bacterial and viral disease. A wide range of rapid diagnostic kits are now commercially available, especially for the high-value horticultural markets.

Intensive agricultural practices are achieving ever more reduced returns at an increasingly detrimental cost to the environment. Genetic engineering offers the potential for improvements in a wide range of agricultural practices but global acceptance must respond to socioeconomic, environmental and safety issues. Are such issues real or have they been excessively exaggerated deliberately by the press? Agricultural biotechnology may not be a panacea for future world food supplies but, if applied correctly and judiciously, it can give real improvements in the quality of life on a global scale.

11

Food and beverage biotechnology

11.1 Introduction

Food production is the largest worldwide industry and, in industrialised nations, the expenditure on food can account for at least 20–30% of household budgets. The food industry has evolved through specialist trades or occupations, e.g. butchers, bakers and confectioners, to national and multi-national organisations involved in the manufacture and distribution of food on a worldwide scale. With the improvement in means of transportation, foods are available on a worldwide basis and developments in food preservation methods give independence for seasonal availability.

In essence, the food industry now serves the function of supplying society with high-quality, wholesome foods all the year round, and at a distance – in time and location – from the place of primary production.

The food chain has its origins in production agriculture, with the planting of the seed or the rearing of animals, and concludes with the utilisation of the food products by the consumer. Apart from fruits and vegetables, most raw food materials, e.g. cereals and meats, will require some degree of processing. The link between the products of the farm and the consumer is the food processing industry, whereby relatively bulky, perishable, raw agricultural products are transformed into shelf-stable, convenient and palatable foods and beverages.

Biotechnology has a long history of practice in food production and processing, and can be viewed as a continuum involving both traditional breeding techniques and the latest techniques based on molecular biology. The new-biotechnology techniques will especially create possibilities of rapidly improving the quantity and quality of food available. Furthermore, the application of these techniques will not result in food which is inherently less safe than that produced by conventional systems. The application of new-biotechnology to produce foods and food ingredients has become a subject of considerable public interest, at consumer, public policy and scientific levels (Chapter 14).

Food biotechnology is concerned with the integration of both modern biological knowledge and techniques and current bioengineering principles in food processing and preservation. This will achieve an elevation of the scientific and technological basis of industrial food processing and preservation to that presently achieved in other advanced biotechnological industries, e.g. antibiotic production. In the next decades, we will witness the integrational optimisation of the production of agricultural materials and their processing into foods and subsequent utilisation.

The challenge is to recognise the potential of biotechnological techniques to fulfil the food requirements of today's society both for developed and developing nations. Food biotechnology encompasses a wide range of options for improved quality, nutrition, safety and preservation of foods. Clearly, no single biotechnological advance will revolutionise the food industry, while economics, customer acceptance and regulatory, rather than scientific, hurdles will have a major influence on the range and spread of food-biotechnology applications. Modern biotechnological techniques will have considerable importance in influencing trends in the food market, namely: cost, preservation, taste, consistency, colour, safety and, above all, health aspects.

The food and beverage industries are very different from the pharmaceutical industry; their products are cost- and marketing-driven rather than technologically driven. Research and development in most of the food and beverage industries is usually less than 1% of sales, is very process-oriented and enjoys little patent protection. Since most food and drink products are high-volume, low-cost items, it is inevitable that market research has become more significant than basic research. Some products such as organic acids, amino acids and gums, now increasingly used by the food and drinks industries, are in the middle price range, while only a few really high-priced products will have a viable future (e.g. sweeteners and flavourings).

The food and beverage industries are high in terms of turnover and labour employed and are very diverse, ranging from small individual producers to giant multinationals.

The impact of biotechnology on the food and beverage industries can be anticipated in two directions:

(1) *agronomic*, i.e. increased plant and animal yields, extended growth range and environments from which the farmers will mainly benefit;

Table 11.1. Biotechnology at all levels of the food chain

Food chain		Potential biotechnological impact
BIOLOGICAL LIVING RAW MATERIALS/ FOOD RAW MATERIALS/FOOD INGREDIENTS	→	*Agronomic*: increased yield; extend geographic and environmental range; all year growing.
		Non-agronomic: increase benefit to processor by lowering the costs of manufacturing operations; keep fresh longer; improve texture and taste; phytoproduction of flavours, colours and other more natural additives, using tissue culture, single cell protein.
	↓	By improving processing and reducing product manufacture costs, e.g. starter cultures, enzyme treatments, genetic engineering of microorganisms, detoxification of food 'toxins', upgrading of waste materials, analytical applications and modification of fatty acids, carbohydrates and proteins.
FOOD PRODUCTS AT THE FACTORY GATE	→	Improve distribution and product quality by inhibiting physical, chemical and microbiological deterioration, introducing less harsh processes and new preservation regimes.
FOOD PRODUCTS AT THE POINT OF CONSUMPTION	→	By ensuring products meet the consumer's expectations of texture, flavour, nutrition, preservation, wholesomeness, and being more natural.
PRODUCTS CONSUMED		

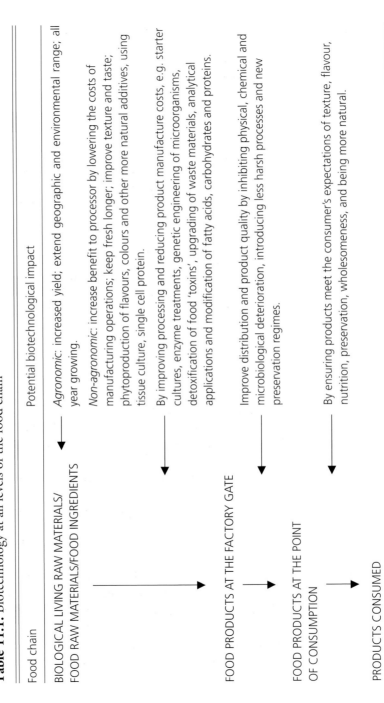

Table 11.2. Some traditional fermented/processed foods and ingredients created by biotechnology methods

Category	Fermented product		
Alcoholic beverages	Beers, wines and spirits		
Food			
Cheese	Sauerkraut	Flavours	Biopolymers
Bread	Soy sauce	Organic acids	Sweeteners
Vinegar	Pickles	Amino acids	Mushrooms
Yoghurt	Enzymes	Vitamins	

(2) *non-agronomic*, i.e. improving plants and microorganisms to provide benefits to the food producer, retailer or consumer (Table 11.1).

New developments in biochemical engineering could also be of advantage to those industries using mechanical (e.g. grinding), physical (e.g. membrane separation, cooking) and chemical (e.g. hydrolysis, salting) methods.

11.2   Food and beverage fermentations

Fermented foods and beverages have a significant role in all societies and result from the action of microorganisms or enzymes on a wide range of agricultural materials, with associated desirable biochemical changes giving significant organoleptic improvements to the final product. As a result of the fermentation process the product is usually more nutritious and more digestible, has improved flavour, and is toxicologically and microbiologically safer.

Fermented foods and beverages derived from plant and animal materials are an accepted and essential part of the diet in almost all parts of the world, involving a wide diversity of raw materials as substrates, using technology from the most primitive to the most advanced, and achieving an astounding range of sensory and textural qualities in the final products. Fermented foods include breads, cheeses, yoghurts, sauerkraut, soy sauce, tempeh and mushrooms, while fermented beverages include alcoholic beers, wines, sake, brandy, whisky and non-alcoholic tea, coffee and cocoa. (For a fuller awareness of this extensive subject, *Fermented Foods of the World: A Dictionary and Guide*, by Campbell-Platt (1989) should be consulted; Table 11.2.) While most of these fermentations remain at the level of village or household arts, others have achieved massive commercial application and play a significant part in most national economies. All such fermentations have been, or remain classified as, indigenous – native to a country or culture – and most were developed before recorded history. However, the very roots of modern biotechnology are to be found in these traditional fermentations. How these fermentations first came about is a question that cannot be completely answered.

Climate and available raw materials have influenced the types of food and beverage fermentations that were geographically developed, and such products continue to form an enduring part of the cultural background of a civilisation. It must be remembered that many of the world's populations are vegetarian, not necessarily by choice but, rather, for mainly economic reasons. While a very important reason for the development of such fermentations was to preserve the basic organic components from spoilage, of equal or greater importance were the resulting changes in organoleptic, physical and nutritional characteristics of the relatively bland starting materials, resulting in products of enhanced flavour, improved vitamin content and, in some vegetable products, a meat-like texture *and* flavour. The nutritional value of these fermentations, in particular to the populations of the developing world, is inestimable and modern fermentation practices (e.g. brewing, cheese making) are providing increased control and consistency of production and, above all, ensuring improved product safety. Food fermentations represent a cornerstone of a civilised society in which raw food materials are processed to make them safe, to have lasting properties and to make them palatable.

For most of these fermentations the procedures were developed in ignorance of the role of microorganisms. The original artisans unwittingly controlled and directed microbial activity by purely empirical methods, but most often achieved consistent end-products. The Egyptians, Sumerians and Babylonians produced alcoholic beverages from barley, and sour-dough bread from rye occurred in Europe in 800 BC, while accounts of fermented dairy products are found in early Sanskrit and Christian works. It is only in relatively recent times that the microbial nature of most of these fermentations has been recognised and, while some fermentations have been shown to have a relatively simple microbiology, others possess a complexity of microbial involvement that may never be fully unravelled.

Fermented foods can be divided into nine groups: beverages, cereal products, dairy products, fish products, fruit and vegetable products, legumes, meat products, starch crop products and miscellaneous products. The relative importance of these fermentations in geographical areas is shown in Table 11.3. These fermentation products represent the largest financial sector of all biotechnologies and a major aspect of gross national product of developed

Table 11.3. Production of classes of fermented foods by geographical region

World production rate	Region	Importance	
		Major	Minor
High	Europe	Dairy, beverage, cereals, meat	Legumes, starch crops
	North America	Beverages, dairy, meat	Fish, legumes, starch crops
	Africa south of Sahara	Starch crops, cereals, beverages	Dairy
Medium	South America	Beverages, dairy	Legumes
	Middle East	Dairy	Legumes, meat
	Indian subcontinent	Cereals, legumes	Meat
	East Asia	Fish, legumes	Dairy
	Southeast Asia	Fish, legumes	Dairy
Low	Oceania	Dairy	Legumes
	North Africa	Dairy	Legumes

From Campbell-Platt (1989).

nations. Almost 90% of all revenues from biotechnology come from the food and beverage sectors. Too often we laud modern biotechnological innovations and overlook the continued presence of the longstanding traditional biotechnology-based industries. However, in almost all sectors of traditional fermentations, new-biotechnology is becoming increasingly exploited.

Some of these fermentations will be examined in more detail and reference made, where relevant, to the impact of modern-biotechnology techniques on their present and future production.

Alcoholic beverages

Alcoholic beverages occur throughout the world in many different forms and tastes. The types of beverages produced in any particular region or country almost entirely reflect the crops grown. Thus, the cooler regions of Europe, Scandinavia, Poland and Russia will produce and consume beers and lagers from barley, while the southern warmer climate of Spain, Greece, Italy and France will have much higher production and consumption of wines derived from grapes. Alcoholic beverages and potable spirit industries worldwide represent one of the most economically stable sectors in modern-day commerce. Demands on economics and the need to increase conversion efficiencies or productivity are all driving forces in the search for new and improved technologies. The main objective is to produce a controlled quantity of alcohol in the liquid to be harvested after the fermentation.

The starting material normally comprises either sugary materials (fruit juices, plant sap, honey) or starchy materials (grains or roots) which need to be hydrolysed to simple sugars before the fermentation (Table 11.4). When these substrates are incubated with suitable microorganisms and allowed to ferment, the end-product is a liquid containing anything from a few per cent up to 16% or more of alcohol, with an acid pH and depleted in nutrients for most contaminating microorganisms; these factors combine to give the product a certain degree of biological stability and safety. The alcoholic beverages can be drunk fresh, but normal practice for many requires a period of storage or ageing, leading in many cases to improved organoleptic properties. Further distillation will increase the alcohol strength and produce spirits of many types, e.g. whisky, brandy, vodka, gin and rum, which can contain 40–50% ethanol (Table 11.5). Cordials and liqueurs are sweetened alcohol distillates derived from fruits, flowers, leaves, etc.

The most regularly used fermenting organism is the yeast *Saccharomyces cerevisiae*, or one of its closely related forms. This yeast is now used for brewing beer and lager, for producing distilled beverages, for many forms of baking, and in most modern wine productions. The present form of *S. cerevisiae* may well have arisen by selection during the evolution of brewing and wine production. It is also most probably the first microbe to have been harnessed for human benefit. The art of making alcoholic beverages by fermentation must have been discovered many times in history as such beverages occur in many different forms the world over. This organism can assimilate and utilise simple sugars such as glucose and fructose and metabolise them to ethanol. It has a high tolerance to ethanol.

S. cerevisiae was the first eukaryote to have its complete genome sequenced, and this will undoubtedly lead to new applications in brewing and baking, together with novel uses. The process details of wine and beer production are briefly examined here since their productions represent major worldwide biotechnological industries.

Wines   Historically, wine is a European drink, and although other parts of the world, e.g. the USA, Australia and South Africa, are now large producers, France, Italy and Germany still produce over half the total world output of approximately 10^{10} litres annually. Historically, the Greeks and Romans preferred wine to beer and, with the spread of Christianity across Europe, wine was used as a symbol of the 'blood of Christ'.

Table 11.4. Substrates for selected alcoholic beverages (non-distilled)

Substrate	Beverage	Country	Saccharifying agent
Starch (barley + other cereals)	Ale	Worldwide (industrial countries)	Barley malt
	Lager		Barley malt
Barley, rye, rice, beet	Kvass	USSR	Barley and rye malt
Millet	Busa	USSR (Crimea)	
	Braga	Roumania	
	Thumba	India	
Rice	Arak	India, SE Asia	
	Busa	Turkistan, SSR	
	Pachwai	India	*Mucor* sp.
	Sake	Japan	*Aspergillus oryzae*
	Sonti	India	
Rice (red)	Ancu	Taiwan	*Rhizopus* sp.
	Hung-Chu	China	
Sorghum	Kaffir beer	Malawi	Sorghum malt
			Aspergillus sp.
			Mucor rouxii
	Merissa	Sudan	*Bacillus* spp.
Sweet potato	Awamori	Japan	Not required since sugar is present in the substrate
Agave spp. (sap)	Pulque	Mexico	
Apple (juice)	Cider	UK, France, N. America	
Grape (juice)	Wine	Temperate: N and S hemispheres	
Honey	Mead	UK	
Pear (juice)	Perry	UK, France	
Palmyra (juice)	'Toddy'	India, SE Asia	
Palm flower-stalk juice	Tuwak	Indonesia	

Table 11.5. Potable alcohol production from sugars or starch-containing raw materials

	Product
Sugar	
Molasses	Rum
	Cognac
Agave	Tequila
Pear	Pear brandy
Cherry	Kirsch
Plums	Slivovice
Starch	
Barley	Whisky
Maize and rye	Bourbon whiskey
Potatoes and barley	Aquavit
Potatoes, rye and wheat	Vodka
Rice	Chinese brandies

Most commercial wines use the wine grape *Vitis vinifera*, and cultivars of this species have been transported throughout the world to establish new wine-producing areas. Soil quality can have an important and subtle effect on the eventual quality of the wine. Red wine is formed when black grapes, are crushed and fermented whole. In contrast, if the skins are removed from black grapes, or when white grapes are used, white wine is the final product. Hundreds of different wines are recognised in the many producing areas of the world. Rosé wine results from some limited contact with the skins of black grapes. Dry wine is the end-product of complete sugar utilisation, while sweet wine will still retain some residual sugars.

Harvesting time of the grapes is judged largely by artisan skills, and the grapes, containing 15–25% sugar, are then crushed mechanically or by treading of feet. The juice (now termed '*must*') is the substrate for the truly biotechnological stage of the production. Since the must will contain many contaminating yeasts and bacteria, it is usual practice to add sulphur dioxide to control or abolish this natural fermentation capacity. In large-scale wine production the must is partially or completely sterilised, inoculated with the desired strain of yeast – *S. cerevisiae* var. *ellipsoideus* – and subjected to controlled fermentation in suitable tanks or bioreactors. The dryness or sweetness of the wine will depend on the degree of sugar conversion, glycerol levels, secondary infections, etc.

Fermentation conditions such as time and temperature will depend on the type of wine desired. After fermentation, the wines are run into storage vats or tankers where the temperature quickly drops, precipitates form and subtle chemical changes take place. Many wines undergo a spontaneous secondary bacterial (*Leuconostoc* spp.) or malolactic fermentation, converting residual malic acid to lactic acid. The final alcoholic content of wines ranges between 10% and 16%.

Modern scientific research now supports the view that moderate wine consumption is associated with lower coronary-heart-disease mortality. As Louis Pasteur stated, 'Wine is the most healthful and most hygienic of beverages'.

Fortified wines, such as sherry, port and vermouth, are wines to which additional alcohol is added after fermentation, raising the alcohol level to about 20%.

Beers   The earliest record of brewing was inscribed in cuneiform characters on clay tablets in Sumeria (present-day Iraq) at least 6000 years ago. However, it is quite possible that primitive forms of brewing existed many thousands of years earlier. Beer can be defined as 'a drink obtained by the alcoholic fermentation of an aqueous extract of germinated cereal with addition of hops'. Beer is a relatively poor medium for bacterial growth, largely owing to its low pH, content of antiseptics such as CO_2, alcohol and hop extracts, and its low temperature of storage. Pathogens cannot live in beer, thus making it safer to drink than water in many countries. Because of its complex biochemical content, beer is almost impossible to analyse. Beers, ales and lagers are produced mostly from starchy cereals such as barley. Additional carbohydrate sources, known as adjuncts, are normally added in varying proportions. In practice, there are five major steps in the manufacture of beers from grains: malting, mashing, fermentation, maturation and finishing (Fig. 11.1).

Malting   Dried barley is soaked or steeped in water and then spread out on the malthouse floor or in revolving drums, where the seeds germinate with the formation of starch-degrading (amylase) and protein-degrading (protease) enzymes. The germinated seeds are then killed by kilning (slow heating to 80°C) while still retaining most of the enzyme activity (*malt*).

Mashing   In this stage the malt is mixed with hot water (55–65°C), and the starches and proteins break down to produce dextrins, maltose and other sugars, protein breakdown products, minerals and other growth factors (the *wort*). This is the medium for the beer fermentation. Hops may be added prior to the fermentation to give characteristic flavour and some antiseptic properties.

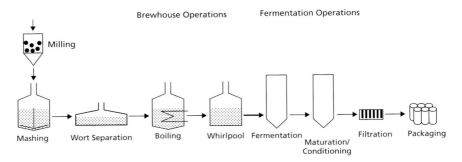

Fig. 11.1 The brewing process, showing the split between the brewhouse and fermentation operations.

Fermentation   The wort is transferred to open-bioreactor systems and inoculated with pure strains of yeast. In Britain, a top-fermenting yeast *Saccharomyces cerevisiae* is used at 20–28°C to produce beers, ales or stouts. In continental Europe, a bottom-fermenting yeast *Saccharomyces uvarum* ferments the wort at a lower temperature (10–15°C) to produce lager.

Maturation and finishing   Beer is usually matured in casks at 0°C for several weeks to improve flavour, settle out the yeasts and remove haze. Bottled or canned beers are usually pasteurised at 60–61°C for 20 minutes. The alcoholic content of beer is usually 4–9%; with ales it is somewhat higher.

While European-type lagers and beers are now produced world-wide, the traditional beer in India and Asia is rice beer and in Africa sorghum beer. Sorghum beer is a very crude material rich in solids and vitamins and is, in fact, a valuable source of nutrition to those who drink it. World annual production of commercial beers is in excess of 750 million hectolitres.

Traditional applied genetics, together with protoplast fusion and recombinant DNA technology, are constantly improving the yeast strains used in these fermentations. In particular, there has been a vast upsurge in genetic engineering knowledge of *S. cerevisiae*. A new commercial brewing yeast has been developed and approved using recombinant DNA techniques.

Coffee, tea and cocoa

In Asia, India, Africa and South America, non-alcoholic fermented beverages are derived from coffee, tea and cocoa plants. These beverages have gained worldwide approval and high commercial value. Tea is derived from the enzymic action released after the crushing of the leaves, while for coffee and cocoa, the pulp surrounding the beans is removed in part by a natural fermentation with bacteria, yeast and fungi, which is critically important for full flavour and aroma development. The dried products, i.e. tea leaves and coffee and cocoa beans, can then be shipped throughout the world and the final beverage formed by the addition of water. Little is known about the exact microbial contribution to these fermentation processes. The processes are still empirical, with little exact science. Huge quantities of these products are consumed worldwide and form the economic basis of several multinational companies.

Dairy products

The manufacture of cultured dairy products represents the second most important fermentation (after the production of alcoholic beverages), accounting for over 20% of fermented foods/drinks produced worldwide. The origin of the development of dairy products such as fermented milk, butter and cheeses is lost in antiquity. Such fermentations are related to areas with high numbers of lactating animals, cows, goats and sheep, and Europe is the major world area of production (Table 11.3). Worldwide, fermented dairy products account for about 10% of all fermented food production. It is now known that these fermentations result largely from the activity of a group of bacteria called 'lactic acid bacteria'. Fermentation by lactic acid bacteria results in preservation and transformation of milk and has been used unknowingly for thousands of years. In the past, these fermentations arose directly from the natural occurrence of lactic acid bacteria, but gradually it was recognised that a portion of a previously successful 'ferment', when added to milk, gave better results. Nowadays, an inoculum (a pure starter culture) of selected bacteria is generally added to the milk to be fermented. The modern worldwide dairy industries owe much to the development of pure starter cultures, good fermentation practices and strict adherence to hygienic protocol.

The lactic acid bacteria can have many beneficial effects in the foods in which they grow, namely:

(1) They have an inhibitory effect (*bacteriocins*) on many undesirable bacteria while they themselves are generally harmless; in this way they preserve the milk.
(2) They produce highly acceptable texture and flavour modifications in the milk.
(3) Reputedly, they have beneficial health effects on intestinal microflora (probiotics).

When growing in milk, these beneficial bacteria break down lactose to lactic acid; however, many other reactions can occur, depending on the composition of the substrate, types of additives and mode of fermentation. These can result in many other metabolites being formed, giving distinctive flavour and appearance to the milk products, e.g. buttermilk, sour cream, yoghurt and the vast range of cheeses.

One of the largest activities of the dairy industry is cheese production. The earliest known reference to cheese is 1800 BC. Cheese is made by separating the casein of milk from the liquid or *whey*. Over 900 individual types of cheese are recognised; yet they could all be prepared from any given batch of milk by proper control of the fermentation and by correct selection of the promoting microorganisms.

The discovery of the role of the animal rennet is believed to have arisen from the use of animal stomachs by nomadic sheep herders for carrying liquids. When milk was transported in this way, it would become heated from the sun, soured by naturally occurring bacteria and contaminated with enzymes (rennet) from the stomach lining. The consequence of this interaction would be the transformation of the milk into solid curds and liquid whey. The curds were then eventually drained, salted and could be used later – an early example of basic food preservation.

In Europe, the Romans were the first to really document this process using sheep or goat's milk. Cow's milk was a very much later innovation. The first industrial production of calf rennet essence or enzymes was in Denmark in 1874. Current world production is now in excess of 30 million litres per year.

Cheese production from milk is essentially a dehydration process in which the milk protein (casein) and fat are concentrated 6–12 times. The common, basic steps in most cheese productions are:

(1) acidification of the milk by the conversion of the sugar lactose into lactic acid by the lactic acid bacteria;
(2) coagulation of the casein by a combination of proteolysis and acidification.

Proteolysis is started by the rennet (chymosin enzyme) (animal or fungal origin) and the coagulated caseins form a gel which entraps any fat present (Fig. 11.2).

The separated curd is cut into blocks, drained and pressed into shapes, matured and made into cheeses. The details of cheese production are very complicated and involve many individual strains of bacteria and, in some cases, filamentous fungi (camembert, blue-cheese), special milks, selected additives and differing process techniques which cannot be covered here.

However, an important recent biotechnological innovation in cheese production has been the use of recombinant DNA techniques for chymosin production *and* commercial use. In the 1960s it became apparent that there

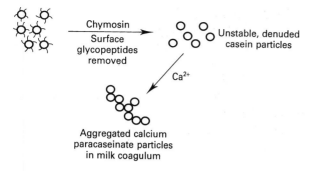

Fig. 11.2 Mode of action of chymosin (rennet).

would be an increasing shortage of animal-derived rennet, and subsequently several substitutes have been developed. At present there are six sources of commercial rennet: three from animals (veal calves, adult cows and pigs) and three fungal sources. The fungal sources are almost identical in function to the animal chymosins and account for approximately a third of world cheese production – particularly in the USA and France. However, they can on occasion, cause yield reductions and poor flavour when compared with animal chymosins.

Within the last decade, genetically modified microorganisms have been produced which can yield identical chymosin to the animal chymosin. Several industrial companies have now produced pure animal-derived chymosin by such methods and these products are now available worldwide. In the UK, at least 95% of chymosin is genetically engineered. The enzyme behaves in exactly the same manner as normal calf chymosin, it has fewer impurities and its activity is more predictable. Contrary to some pessimistic forecasts, recombinant chymosin has been well received by the public and also by the Vegetarian Society. Expert tasters cannot detect any difference between cheeses made using recombinant chymosin and calf chymosin. Its commercial success is ensured. The production of calf chymosin by genetically modified microorganisms is shown in Fig. 11.3.

The flavour of raw cheese, such as Cheddar, is bland and the texture rubbery. It is the period of ripening or maturation, when other microorganisms such as bacteria and fungi can have pronounced effects, that causes the development of distinctive flavours and aromas as well as major textural changes (Table 11.6). World cheese markets now exceed $26 000 million annually.

The second major group of dairy products are the yoghurts. They are major foods consumed worldwide and represent one of the fastest growing food products in the food industry. Claims are now being made that live

Table 11.6. Principal types of cheeses

Unripened cheeses
Low fat (cottage cheese)
High fat (cream cheese)

Ripened cheeses
Hard cheese (internal ripening)
   Ripened by bacteria (Cheddar, and Swiss cheese)
   Ripened by mould (Roquefort and other blue cheeses)
Soft cheeses (ripening proceeds from outside)
   Ripened by bacteria (Limburger)
   Ripened by bacteria and moulds (Camembert)

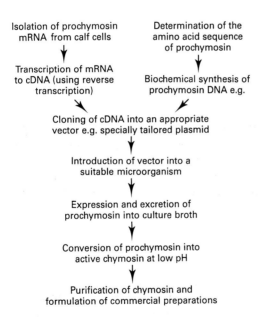

Fig. 11.3   Production of calf chymosin by genetically modified microorganisms.

yoghurt bacteria can become established in the human gut with benefits to the digestive and other systems. This growing field of *probiotics* is still to be definitively proved in humans but is increasingly being viewed as an important future area of medical advance.

Traditionally, yoghurt is fermented whole milk; the process uses a mixed culture of *Lactobacillus bulgaricus* and *Streptococcus thermophilus*. The characteristic flavour compound, acetaldehyde, is produced by *Lb. bulgaricus* while

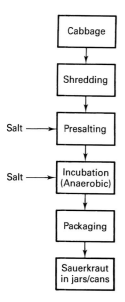

Fig. 11.4 The production of sauerkraut.

the *Strep. thermophilus* generates the fresh acid taste by the conversion of lactose to lactic acid. Both bacteria produce extracellular polymers that give the characteristic viscosity of the product. Incubation is at 30°C or 45°C. Set yoghurt is packed into the container after inoculation and allowed to ferment in the container. Frozen yoghurt is gaining increasing popularity as an alternative for ice cream.

Vegetable fermentations

In various ways throughout the world, fruits and vegetables can be preserved using salt and acid – the acid being derived largely from bacteria in the form of lactic acid. Of particular western interest is the fermentation preservation of cabbage to give sauerkraut and the pickling of cucumbers and olives.

In sauerkraut production, shredded cabbage is packed anaerobically with salt, the salt reducing the water activity and promoting the leakage of sugars from the cabbage leaves (Fig. 11.4). Subsequently, lactic acid bacteria proliferate, releasing lactic acid, lowering the pH and preventing the growth of putrefying bacteria. Accurate control of temperature (7.5°C), salt concentration (2.25%) and the anaerobic state will produce excellent, long-lasting sauerkraut – a nutritious, tasteful food. Large-scale production of sauerkraut can be traced back in Germany to the year AD 800. Much research is in progress to produce sauerkraut with lower salt concentrations.

In cucumber and olive fermentations, especially in Greece and Spain, the fermentations are carried out at much higher salt concentrations (5–8%) and the microbial sequences are relatively similar to sauerkraut fermentation.

Cereal products

In almost all parts of the world, cereals are produced and are the main class of food consumed by man; a considerable proportion of these cereals will be fermented into solid foods or into alcoholic beverages.

Bread in its many local forms is the principal fermented cereal product and has been known since Roman times. The bread market is worth at least $3 billion a year worldwide. In Europe, wheat and rye are two widely used cereal flours and are usually mixed with water or milk, salt, fat, sugar and other varied ingredients, together with the yeast *Saccharomyces cerevisiae*. As the fermentation proceeds, the dough rises owing to the formation of CO_2. The expansion and stretching of the dough, particularly with wheat, is due to the unique extensible and elastic protein gluten. In this way the dough rises and retains its shape on oven baking.

Early forms of bread were unleavened and similar to modern naan breads. It is believed that contamination of such flat-bread mixtures by natural yeasts yielded the first 'risen' breads, which were much more palatable. The Romans are believed to have introduced leavened bread to western Europe.

Bread texture is affected by fats, emulsifiers and oxidising agents while the speed of bread making (of commercial importance) is affected by fats, oxidising and reducing agents and soya flour. While the yeast enzymes have an important role, additional enzymes, e.g. amylases, are added to assist mixing, fermentation, baking and eventual storage characteristics of the bread. Modern biotechnology will increasingly supply improved enzymes to bring even greater control over this complex process.

Overall, the fermentation achieves three primary objectives: leavening (CO_2 production), flavour development and texture changes in the dough. At the end of the fermentation process the risen dough is baked in an oven, giving a final product which is free of living microorganisms and which has an extended shelf-life.

Modern applied genetics seeks always to improve the quality of the yeast organism, leading to improved activity, better flavour and improved texture of the product. A genetically engineered *Saccharomyces cerevisiae* with improved fermentation properties has been produced and has passed all regulatory requirements for safety. However, as yet, the producer company has not put it into commercial operation!

In other parts of the world, *sourdough breads* use yeast *Candida milleri* and *Lactobacillus sanfrancisco* for the fermentation stage, while *Streptococcus* and *Pediococcus* species are used in the Indian subcontinent to ferment mixtures of cereal and legume flours to produce *idli* and *poppadoms*. Rice is widely used in Asia during legume and fish fermentations. In South America, *corn bread* from the cereal maize is a staple food.

New strains of baking yeasts are regularly being developed (not yet by recombinant DNA technology) and most research is directed into improving the technology of bread making and the preservation of the final product, especially by packaging innovations.

Legume fermentations

The soya bean *Glycine max* is the main legume used for fermentation, and products derived are of particular importance in diets in East Asia, Southeast Asia and India. Fermentation will improve digestibility of the beans by breaking down anti-nutritional factors and compounds that cause flatulence in the intestine. In Indonesia, cooked soya beans are fermented with the fungus *Rhizopus oligosporus* and the product, tempeh, fried in oil and eaten as a snack or in soups. Over 250 000 people are involved in the production of tempeh in Indonesia. There is a growing interest in this product in Europe and the USA.

The major fermentation of soya beans is in the production of *soy sauce* and *miso*. The production of soy sauce has three phases: the *koji*, the *moromi* and *maturation*. The koji is a solid-substrate fermentation in which cooked soya beans and wheat flour are fermented with *Aspergillus oryzae* to break down starches, proteins and pectins. The moromi is a liquid/slurry fermentation under anaerobic conditions, with *Candida* and *Pediococcus* as the fermentation agents. Maturation gives the final full-flavour spectrum.

Table 11.7 gives details of Japanese consumptions of soy sauce and related soya bean-fermented products. The Asiatic countries enjoy a rich range of legume- and rice-fermented products with high annual per-capita consumption.

In all of the discussed food and beverage fermentations, specific microorganisms play an indispensable function in achieving the final product. Starter cultures are now used in all of these fermentations and bring control and

Table 11.7. Per capita annual consumption of fermented foods prepared from Aspergillus moulds in Japan (1981)

Food	Per capita/yeast	Total production/year
1 Soy sauce	10.1 l	1 200 000 kl
2 Miso	4.9 kg	572 000 t
3 Sake	12.3 l	1 445 000 kl
4 Mirin	0.6 l	260 000 kl
5 Shochu	2.2 l	30 000 kl
6 Rice vinegar	2.5 l	305 000 kl
Note:		
Beer		4 656 000 kl
Whisky and other foreign alcoholic beverages	3.7 l	445 000 kl

Note: Japanese population 117 850 000 (1 October 1981).
From Yokotsuka (1985).

greater uniformity to the end-product(s). In most processes the microorganisms become part of the food and are consumed intact. In others e.g. wine, beer, vinegar and soy sauce, the cells are removed by filtration or centrifugation to eliminate turbidity.

11.3   Enzymes and food processing

Enzymes are indispensable in modern food processing technology. Enzymes are an essential part of most food and beverage fermentations and, while most of the enzymes will be derived from participating microorganisms, increasingly processes are being improved by the direct addition of exogenous enzymes (Table 11.8). There will be an increasing production of food enzymes using rDNA biotechnology. Chymosin has been the front runner for this new technology and its use now exceeds 80% of the market in the USA and Canada. The accepted use of chymosin or other enzymes by rDNA technology is based on the following: enzyme preparations are free of any bioprocessing and purification steps and viable-rDNA biotechnology-driven microorganisms are not present in the final preparation. Improvements are increasingly apparent in enzyme availability, purity and cost which will benefit and improve the quality of foods available to consumers. Examples close to commercialisation include lactase for lactose hydrolysis, α-amylase and amyloglucosidase

Table 11.8. Use of enzymes in food processing

Industry	Enzymes used	Expenditure (US $ million)
Brewing	α-amylase, β-amylase, protease, papain, amyloglucosidase, xylanase	30
Dairy	Animal/microbial chymosins, lactase, lipase, lysozyme	90
Baking	α-amylase, xylanase, protease, phospholipase A and D, lipoxygenase	20
Fruit and vegetable processing	Pectinesterase, polygalacturanase, pectin lyase, hemicellulases	18
Starch and sugar	α-amylase, β-amylase, glucoamylase, xylanase, pullulanase, isomerase, oligoamylases	120

for high-fructose corn syrup, and acetolactate decarboxylase for beer aging and diacetyl reduction.

The role of exogenous enzymes in facilitating or even replacing mechanical processes is well demonstrated in fruit and vegetable processing, while in industrial starch transformation, chemical processing has yielded almost completely to enzyme processing.

A major development which will revolutionise the use of enzymes in the food industry involves the near elimination of water from enzyme reaction media. Thus, hydrolytic enzymes can be reversed so that, with no metabolic energy input, the same enzymes that degrade biomolecules can now synthesise them. A wide range of food-related compounds have now been produced by this novel approach and include polyglycerol esters (emulsifiers), chiral-flavour esters and oligopeptides, and structural polymers.

The new concept of protein engineering will facilitate the design or alteration of food enzymes at a molecular level, allowing minor modifications or the design of completely novel enzyme catalysts. An important application has involved the enzyme phospholipase A2, currently used as a food emulsifier. There is little doubt that the process of protein engineering coupled to gene cloning technology will be extensively applied to many enzymes used in food processing, allowing greater accuracy and selectivity of action.

Enzymes will also be extensively used in the design of novel and functional foods. Particularly in Japan, there has been considerable research into oligosaccharides for insulin-low calorie response, designer fats and special food-fibre

Table 11.9. Traditional and alternative sweeteners

Product	Relative sweetness
Sucrose	1.0
55% HFCS	1.4
Cyclamate	50
Aspartame	150
Saccharin	300
Thaumatin	3000

ingredients. Much effort is now being directed into the role of nutrition and the ageing process. The affluent, ageing populations of the West will wholeheartedly support such research efforts!

11.4 Sweeteners

In most societies there is a considerable need for sweeteners to accompany food intake. The annual consumption of sweeteners in the USA and Europe is approximately 57 kg of sucrose equivalent per capita. Up to the late 1960s, sweeteners were mainly cane and beet sugar – sucrose. In the 1970s, enzyme technology created a new class of sweeteners derived from starch (see Chapter 5: high-fructose syrups). Saccharin, which is chemically derived, has been widely used as a sweetener for many years but is now being increasingly challenged by new, natural, low-calorific sweeteners, while biotechnological methods have been used to develop one of the most important additions to this market – aspartame. Aspartame (tradename Nutra-sweet) is used extensively in many low-calorie 'diet' soft drinks. Thaumatin, a protein extracted from berries of the plant *Thaumatococcus danielli*, is the sweetest compound known (Table 11.9). It is marketed extensively in Japan and now Europe and considerable effort is being made to produce the protein in genetically engineered microorganisms.

Sweeteners find extensive markets and applications in soft drinks, confectionery, jams and jellies, ice cream, canning, baking, fermentation, pickles and sauces, and meat products – truly an immense market that will benefit from biotechnological innovations.

The most expensive component in the synthesis of aspartame is the amino acid phenylalanine, which is now produced on a large scale by fermentation methods. Extensive toxicological studies were necessary before aspartame was permitted to be marketed. All new biotechnologically derived food products must undergo a programme of regulatory approval similar to that demanded for new pharmaceuticals. Approval for aspartame took 10 years.

11.5   Food wastes

Wastes from food and drinks industries are becoming an increasing problem, particularly to large production centres, because of increasingly strict legislation on the dumping of high-BOD (biological oxygen demand) wastes (Chapter 9). Much effort is now being made to use such organic wastes to generate valuable by-products, while also achieving active waste removal. There is a large market for biological waste-treatment systems.

11.6   Miscellaneous microbial-derived food products

These products are derived from microbial fermentations and are used as ingredients in food production.

Vinegar

Vinegar is an aqueous solution containing at least 4% acetic acid and small amounts of esters, sugars, alcohol and salts. It is usually derived from wine, malt or apple cider. The fermenting bacteria are normally species of *Acetobacter*. It is widely used as an acidulant and flavouring compound in processed liquid foods such as sauces and ketchups.

Organic acids

Citric acid is widely used in the food-related industries in fruit drinks, confectionery, jams, preserved fruits, etc. Over 100 000 tonnes of citric acid are manufactured annually by fermentation processes involving the fungus *Aspergillus niger* and molasses as substrate. The fermentation can be as static, liquid, surface cultures in trays, or in deep-tank, large-scale bioreactors. Citric acid is used in foods to enhance the flavour, to prevent oxidation and browning, and as a preservative. Lactic acid can be produced by fermentation (40%) or by chemical synthesis (60%) and is used largely as an acidulant. Other organic acids include gluconic and itaconic acids.

Table 11.10. Worldwide production of amino acids

Production (tonnes per year)	Amino acid	Preferred production method	Main use
800 000	L-glutamic acid	Fermentation	Flavour enhancer
350 000	L-lysine	Fermentation	Feed additive
350 000	D, L-methionine	Chemical synthesis	Feed additive
10 000	L-aspartate	Enzymatic catalysis	Aspartame
10 000	L-phenylalanine	Fermentation	Aspartame
15 000	L-threonine	Fermentation	Feed additive
10 000	Glycine	Chemical synthesis	Food additives, sweeteners
10 000	L-cysteine	Reduction of cystine	Food additives

From Eggeling, Pfefferle and Sahm (2001).

Amino acids and vitamins

Amino acids are widely used in the food and beverage industries as flavour enhancers, as seasonings, or as nutritional additives. World production levels for food use are in excess of 1.6 million tonnes per year, with Japan commanding a major proportion of the US$2 billion market. Glutamic acid and lysine are two amino acids produced by fermentation processes involving the bacteria *Corynebacterium glutamicum* and *Brevibacterium flavum* respectively (Table 11.10). Extensive mutant selection has produced microorganisms that overproduce these primary metabolites. DNA technology will further improve the production capabilities. Vitamins are usually used as dietary supplements. However, vitamin C (ascorbic acid) is used as a food ingredient; annual production is about 40 000 tonnes. Several microorganisms can be used in the production processes.

Amino acids and vitamins are now considered as classified products in biotechnology and, for their continued development, there must be regular improvements in the processes, the establishment of new processes, and constant reappraisal of the producer microorganisms.

Polysaccharides

Extracellular microbial polysaccharides are produced copiously by many microorganisms and have been used in foods to enhance thickening and to form gels. They can stabilise food structure and improve appearance and palatability. The bacterial species mainly used are *Pseudomonas* spp. (xanthan gums) and *Leuconostoc mesenteroides* (dextrans). Species of *Acetobacter* can produce cellulose, which forms the basis of certain oriental foods.

Flavours/flavour enhancers

The best-known flavour or sensory enhancer is monosodium glutamate, now largely made by fermentation using natural or engineered microorganisms. Enzymatic degradation of yeast RNA can produce nucleotide derivatives which are powerful flavour enhancers for meat. The current world market for food flavours is about $2.0 billion and increasing. Biotechnology will have a profound influence on this market using gene manipulation and improved enzyme procedures.

11.7   Rapid diagnostics

It is a major requirement of all food processes to supply a product that is free of dangerous microbial toxins. A wide array of traditional, time-consuming procedures have routinely been applied to identify, control, reduce or remove such contaminants. Major food pathogens include *Listeria, Salmonella and Campylobacter*, while the bacterial endotoxins and the fungal mycotoxins are the principal toxins considered.

Developments in biotechnology now permit a complete reshaping of many of these testing protocols by the application of antibody-detection systems and DNA and RNA probe technology. These procedures are much shorter in time, generally cheaper, and often do not need highly skilled operators. By means of these new technologies there will be major improvements in safety standards in the food supply.

The use of immunoassays in the food industry is a recent development but is rapidly becoming an accepted analytical tool. The enzyme-linked immunosorbent assay (ELISA) (Chapter 10), based on a 96-well micro-titration plate, is the most widely used format by the food scientist. It is extremely versatile in that a wide range of handling methods can be used, from manual operation to completely automated assays. Time and labour savings offered by ELISAs over conventional assays can be considerable. The detection of *Salmonella* bacteria in foods is a very complex procedure and can take up to 5 days using traditional enrichment procedures. By means of immunoassay procedures, this can be as little as 1 day. Similarly, the mycotoxin aflatoxin requires many hours of extraction, purification and concentration for accurate traditional chemical identification. However, using affinity columns containing the specific antibodies to the toxin, the whole process of extraction and quantification can be carried out within 30 minutes.

Food immunoassay procedures are now available for many potential food analytes, e.g. trace residues, mycotoxins, antibiotics, hormones and bacterial toxins. With the increased development and availability of such diagnostic procedures in user-friendly kit form, new options will be available for food safety control which will achieve obvious benefits to manufacturer, consumer and regulatory authorities.

11.8   Bioprocess technology

In food biotechnology, fermentation is the main means of producing a wide range of products; the basic concepts of bioprocess technology have been considered in Chapter 4. Improved bioprocess technology in food production will increase productivity, lower costs, improve nutrition and reduce environmental damage presently occurring in many food processes.

11.9   Public acceptance and safety of new biotechnology foods

The public, to some extent, have a *negative* attitude to excessive manipulation of foods and demonstrate some hostility, in particular, to genetic engineering of foodstuffs. This highly controversial topic is discussed in much more detail in Chapter 14.

The food industry is highly conservative and slow to welcome technological change. The ultimate full acceptance of new biotechnology in the food sector will depend on many interacting factors, e.g. economics, consumer acceptance, regulatory procedures, and the types of technology. Biotechnology has a great ability to increase productivity by decreasing costs per unit of output or by increasing yields per unit of output. Biotechnology will increase the vertical integration of agriculture and the food industry. At present, new biotechnology is having a greater impact in developed nations. It is to be hoped that these new approaches can also be brought to the advantage of the developing nations, where food needs are greatest.

As with all advances in food technology, it must always be remembered that food is to be eaten and that it must be good to eat.

12

Protection of biotechnological inventions

The British National Economic Development Office has projected that the sales worldwide from new biotechnology could exceed £60 billion per annum by early this century. This will be derived from a wide range of biotechnology-based products and processes which have evolved, in most cases, from many years of expensive research and development. How can such biotechnology products and processes be protected and the due financial profits returned to the rightful inventors and industrial developers? Inventors in the area of biotechnology can be protected by way of different titles of protection, including patents for invention, plant breeders' rights and trade secrets. In the context of biotechnology inventions can be in the form of products or processes.

Products These can be considered *either* as living entities of natural or artificial origin, e.g animals, plants and microorganisms, cell lines, organelles, plasmids and DNA sequences, or as naturally occurring substances – primary or secondary – derived from living systems.

Processes These can include those of isolation, cultivation, multiplication, purification and bioconversion. Such processes can be involved in: the isolation or the creation of the above products, e.g. antibiotic production; the production of substances through bioconversion of products, e.g. enzymatic conversion of sugar to alcohol; or the use of the products for any purpose, e.g. monoclonal antibodies used for analysis or diagnosis, or microbes used for biocontrol of pathogens.

12.1   Patent protection

What is a patent? A patent is a legal right which owes its existence to a granting act by a governmental administrative authority, i.e. a patent office. The patent office must be certain that the patent meets three critical criteria:

(1) *Novelty*. It has not been done before or even talked about in public meetings.
(2) *Utility*. It has a useful purpose. For instance, a gene is not patentable on its own right but should be related to a product.
(3) *Enablement*. It can be repeated by someone.

With the granting of the patent, the holder or patentee is given the right to exclude, for a limited time period, all others within the territory of application of the patent for commercial utilisation of the patent invention. In return for this monopoly situation, the patentee discloses the details of the invention to the public so that, at the end of the monopoly period, the invention may be worked freely by the public (i.e. other competitors). To obtain patent rights in, for example, Europe, the USA and Japan, the patent application must be made in each country. Such multiple applications can be very expensive and restricting. Some parts of the world still do not have legally installed patent systems and may attempt to exploit published patents without any financial return to the patentee.

After the patent application has been scrutinised and granted, the patent is in the form of a letter patent which, *inter alia*, contains the name of the inventor, the name of the patentee (if different), a description of the patent and the relevant claims. Patents can be granted for inventions that:

(1) are novel,
(2) involve an inventive step,
(3) can lead to industrial application,
(4) are seen to be properly disclosed in the patent specification.

Unlike other fields of technology, inventions in biotechnology most often relate to living materials, which can raise some unique difficulties in their legal protection. Problems can arise as to how to describe an invention relating to living material for the purpose of obtaining patent protection and, most basically, whether living matter *should* be protectable under traditional schemes of industrial property protection and, if so, what range of protection should be given to such material. For example, the National Institute of Health, in

USA, was refused patent rights on segments of DNA isolated from the human genome (Chapter 8).

In this context the difference between discovery (not patentable) and invention for a biotechnological substance has been highlighted by the European Patent Office:

> To find a substance freely occurring in nature is . . . mere discovery and
> therefore unpatentable. However, if a substance found in nature has first to be
> isolated from its surroundings and a process for obtaining it is developed, that
> process is patentable. Moreover, if the substance can be properly characterised,
> either by its chemical structure, by the process by which it is obtained or by
> other parameters and if it is 'new' in the absolute sense of having no previous
> recognised existence, then the substance *per se* may be patentable.

From a microorganism standpoint the claim that a human-made, genetically engineered *Pseudomonas* bacterium was capable of breaking down multiple components of crude oil (developed by Chakrabarty in the USA for oil-spill biodegradation) was 'not to a hitherto unknown natural phenomenon, but to a non-naturally occurring manufacture or composition of matter – a product of human ingenuity having distinctional name, character and use'. The patent claim was for a new bacterium which had potential for significant industrial use and which had different characteristics from any found in nature, thereby qualifying this bacterium as a patentable subject – it was *not* nature's handiwork but that of the patentee. This patent award has significantly improved future success for genetically engineered organisms, which are now coming forward in ever-increasing numbers for patent consideration.

Another interesting example for patent consideration was the *onco-mouse* – a mouse genetically manipulated so that it was more predisposed to detect carcinogens than an ordinary mouse. The European Patent Convention excludes inventions 'in respect of plant or animal varieties or essentially biological processes for the production of plants or animals; this provision does not apply to microbiological processes or the products thereof'. Much of biotechnology is, however, microbiological and, therefore, prima facie patentable. Macrobiological processes involving plants and animals are excluded. A patent was awarded for the onco-mouse on the narrowest of grounds in part because the process of production could not occur in nature (as the mice would not have existed had it not been for the microbiological gene-insertion process into the mouse DNA) and, therefore, the process was not essentially biological.

The oncomouse is more susceptible to developing tumours, which makes it valuable for studying cancer and the potential therapeutic benefit from drugs that could be used to treat cancer.

Table 12.1. Benefits and disadvantages of the patent system

Benefits	Disadvantages
(1) The patent holder retains an absolute monopoly on the product or process for the period of patent (up to 20 years in some cases).	(1) Knowledge is in public domain following expiry and could be valuable to competitors.
(2) Administration of patent maintenance, once it has been obtained, is relatively easy.	(2) Litigation can be expensive.
	(3) Problems of lack of harmonisation of patent laws and other trading blocks not covered by patent could tolerate misuse.

In Europe, there continues to be much vocal opposition to animal and human gene patenting, and to biotechnology in general. In the USA, the prospect for patenting animals is less daunting and several transgenic animals have, so far, been patented. However, advancements in this area of biotechnology will continue to face strong opposition, more often from religious coalitions who believe that altering or creating new life forms is 'a revolt against the sovereignty of God and an attempt to be God'. Since these currently approved animal patents are for medical benefits, there should be a distinction made between 'playing God' and 'playing doctor'. The fundamental policy behind the granting of patents is not the ownership of property rights but, rather, the encouragement of the development of technology and innovations.

Patent laws are remarkably complex and tend to vary between different parts of the world. It is a legal minefield but necessary to ensure the just financial returns for those who invest heavily in biotechnological research and development, without which there would be no forward advance in the many dimensions of biotechnology. The benefits and disadvantages of patents are shown in Table 12.1. Whether an invention should be patented must be a commercial decision, assisted by legal advice and involving a good level of business and common sense, together with an awareness of the main alternative to patenting – namely, secrecy. Only a very small percentage of patents will be real winners achieving high financial returns.

Patenting of a new effective drug allows the manufacturer to sell the drug at a good profit for the duration of the patent without competition. Once the

Table 12.2. Benefits and disadvantages of the trade secret system

Benefits	Disadvantages
(1) Knowledge of the system is not public and so is not available to competitors.	(1) Someone else could have same idea and exploit it.
(2) There is no time limit on the available protection.	(2) Some countries may not recognise the protection of confidential information.
	(3) In-house procedures need to be elaborate, time consuming and tedious.
	(4) The enforcement of confidentiality procedures can be problematic.

drug comes 'off patent' it can then be manufactured by others as a 'generic' and profit margins drop dramatically.

12.2   Trade secrets

Many biotechnology companies prefer to use trade secrets to protect their products or processes rather than to apply for patents. The forms of information that can be protected include, for example, hybridoma cell lines for monoclonal antibody production; ideas, formula and production details; and experimental procedures. In the citric acid industry, production strains and details of medium design and formulation are highly confidential and full details are only known by a few employees.

Undoubtedly the best-kept trade secret in the world is the formula for Coca-Cola. The formula is kept in a bank in Atlanta, USA, and only five people in the world are said to know the formula. The formula has remained a secret for over 100 years and has allowed a huge commercial empire to develop and continue.

Such trade secrets can only be protected if they are kept confidential, and a company needs to operate appropriate measures to retain confidential information within the company. Contracts of employment can include confidentiality clauses, and may even restrict an employee from later working for a competitor. In many biotechnology companies such as the whisky industry, this has long been common practice. The benefits and disadvantages of proceeding by the trade secrets route are shown in Table 12.2.

12.3   Plant breeders' rights

Under various national and international agreements and acts, plant varieties are protected by giving the plant breeders limited monopoly rights over the varieties they have created by way of a registration system for plant varieties. Those who use the seeds or plants will, by right, pay a royalty to the breeder. However, there is an important provision that the farmers can retain a proportion of the seeds of a crop for re-planting. Purchasers can also use the variety to develop new varieties, which the purchaser will own the rights to – not the creator of the original variety. The advent of recombinant DNA technology, which can permit the creation of large numbers of new varieties much more easily and quickly than traditional genetic methods, will undoubtedly undermine the protection conferred by plant-variety rights. Intensive legal discussions are now in progress in nations with high commitment to plant genetic-engineering methodology.

13

Safety in biotechnology

13.1   Introduction

In previous chapters the many applications of biotechnology can be divided into the traditional domains of fermentation for the production of various potable beverages, bread, cheese, organic acids, antibiotics and waste treatment, and the new biotechnologies, including production and use of genetically modified organisms for the large-scale production of vaccines, therapeutic proteins and other health products, together with the use of hybridomas for the production of monoclonal antibodies for diagnostic and therapeutic end-points. As such, biotechnology spans a vast range of industrial activities, and considerations of biosafety can potentially encompass activities within the research laboratory, the process plant, the final product and, in many cases, the environment. The term 'biosafety' has evolved as a new area of corporate activity created as an inevitable response generated by an expanding biotechnology industry and its increasing influence upon may aspects of commercial and public life. In particular, the many public issues recently generated, especially in Europe, concerning genetically modified crop trials have done much to raise the profile of this subject.

In all biotechnology processes, however, safety is of paramount importance. Table 13.1 lists the main areas of consideration for safety aspects in biotechnology.

Table 13.1. Safety considerations in biotechnology

Pathogenicity: potential ability of living organisms and viruses (natural and genetically engineered) to infect humans, animals and plants and to cause disease

Toxicity and allergy associated with microbial production

Other medically relevant effects: increasing the environmental pool of antibiotic-resistant microorganisms

Problems associated with the disposal of spent microbial biomass and the purification of effluents from biotechnological processes

Safety aspects associated with contamination, infection or mutation of process strains

Safety aspects associated with the industrial use of microorganisms containing *in vitro* recombinant DNA

Table 13.2. Hazard and risk determination

Hazard	Risk
Qualitative	Quantitative, potentially
Concerned with identification of the hazard and causes	Concerned with consequences
Also called 'what-if?'	Also called 'risk analysis', 'risk assessment', 'quantitative risk assessment'
Best identified by teams	Best identified singly or in small groups

13.2   Concepts of hazard and risk

Essential to the understanding of biosafety are the recognition and appreciation of the terms 'hazard' and 'risk'. In the context of health and safety, 'hazard' can be a substance, object or situation with a potential for an accident or damage, and 'risk' is the likelihood that this will occur (Table 13.2). Simply put, a hazard is something with the potential to cause harm, while risk defines the chance of an individual or the environment being harmed by the hazard. Biosafety standards are now based on international technical state-of-the-art and relevant legislation which aims to prevent risk to human health and the environment resulting from activities involving biological agents.

Table 13.3. Risk assessment

Elucidate the capacity of the microorganism to have an adverse effect on humans or the environment.
Establish the probability that microorganisms might escape, either accidentally or inadvertently, from the production process system.
Evaluate the safety of the desired products and the methods for handling by-products.

13.3   Problems of organism pathogenicity

Many microorganisms can infect humans, animals and plants and cause disease. Successful establishment of disease results from interactions between the host and the causal organism. Many factors are involved, only a few of which are well understood.

Most microorganisms used by industry are harmless and many are indeed used directly for the production of human or animal foods. Many such examples have been discussed elsewhere in this book and include yeasts, filamentous fungi and many bacteria. Their safety is well documented from long associations lasting up to hundreds of years. Only a small number of potentially dangerous microorganisms have been used by industry in the manufacture of vaccines or diagnostic reagents, e.g. *Bordetella pertussis* (whooping cough), *Mycobacterium tuberculosis* (tuberculosis) and the virus of foot-and-mouth disease. Stringent containment practices have been the norm when these microorganisms are used.

In recent years there have been many scientific advances permitting alterations to the genetic make-up of microorganisms. Recombinant DNA techniques have been the most successful but have also been the cause of much concern to the public (Chapter 14). However, this natural anxiety has been ameliorated by several compelling lines of evidence:

(1) Risk-assessment studies have failed to demonstrate that host cells can acquire novel hazardous properties from DNA donor cells (Table 13.3).
(2) More rigorous evaluation of existing information concerning basic immunology, pathogenicity and infectious disease processes has led to relaxation of containment specifications previously set down.
(3) Considerable experimentation has shown no observable hazard.

However, care must always be adopted when using recombinant DNA molecules (see also Chapter 3). There have been suggestions made for the need of international protocols for the testing and shipment of genetically modified organisms. Existing international mechanisms are already dealing effectively with such potential safety issues connected with genetic engineering. While there is a vast amount of evidence that the application of genetic engineering is safe and that the biotechnological developments with plants and animals are being applied responsibly and safely, there are still some bodies of opinion that seek draconian biosafety protocols based on conjectured potential consequences of genetic engineering. Never has a new technology been more thoroughly scientifically scrutinised than in these new areas of biotechnology. Many of the opponents use inflammatory and totally unscientific reasoning in their attempts to derail this potentially valuable technology. Scientific research on safety aspects of this technology will continue to be an important and continuing issue.

The European Federation of Biotechnology Working Party on Biosafety has now been established to provide recommendations on safety aspects of biotechnology with respect to the environment, the public, personnel and product, to include:

- identifying and monitoring hazards associated with various applications in biotechnology;
- assessing and quantifying risks;
- providing an international platform for issues related to safety in biotechnology;
- producing statements and recommendations (based on science and technology);
- identifying areas of insufficient knowledge and inadequate technology with respect to safety in biotechnology and proposing research and development in such areas;
- assisting in the implementation of the recommendations and guidelines in biotechnology.

A classification of the degree of potential hazard of microorganisms has been drawn up by the European Federation of Biotechnology (Table 13.4). Class 5 contains those microorganisms that present risks only to the environment, particularly to animals and plants.

13.4   Problems of biologically active biotechnology products

Vaccines and antibiotics are obvious examples of biologically active products, and care must be taken to prevent their indiscriminate dispersal. Contaminants

Table 13.4. Classification of microorganisms according to pathogenicity

Class 1
Microorganisms that have never been identified as causative agents of disease in man and which offer no threat to the environment.

Class 2
Microorganisms that may cause human disease and which might, therefore, offer a hazard to laboratory workers. They are unlikely to spread in the environment. Prophylactics are available and treatment is effective.

Class 3
Microorganisms that offer a severe threat to the health of laboratory workers but a comparatively small risk to the population at large. Prophylactics are available and treatment is effective.

Class 4
Microorganisms that cause severe illness in humans and offer a serious hazard to laboratory workers and to people at large. In general, effective prophylactics are not available and no effective treatment is known.

Class 5
Microorganisms that offer a more severe threat to the environment than to people. They may be responsible for heavy economic losses. National and international lists and regulations concerning these microorganisms are already in existence in contexts other than biotechnology (e.g. for phytosanitary purposes).

in otherwise safe processes may produce toxic molecules that could become incorporated into final products, leading to food poisoning. Allergenic reactions to produce formulations must also be guarded against. Over-use of antibiotics in agriculture could lead to carry-over into human foods, resulting in possible development of antibiotic resistance in human disease organisms. Many countries now restrict the use of antibiotics in agriculture.

When properly practised, biotechnology is safe and the benefits deriving from biotechnological innovations will surely lead to major improvements in the health and well-being of the world's population. However, biotechnology must always be subjected to sound regulations for its successful application. The potential risks of biotechnology are manageable, and regulations have been constructed for that management.

13.5   Biowarfare and bioterrorism

There is a growing worldwide concern that pathogenic microorganisms may be used in acts of urban terrorism. All major nations have, at some time, run major research programmes on biological warfare. While the use of bioweapons is prohibited under the Biological and Toxic Weapon Convention, there can be no doubt that some rogue nations have not subscribed to this ban and, while biowarfare is unlikely, the availability of such potential pathogenic bioagents could lead to acts of bioterrorism.

Potential biological agents have been assigned to three categories (Centre for Disease Control, Atlanta, USA):

category A   agents include the most serious – smallpox, anthrax, plague, botulism, tularaemia and viral haemorrhagic fevers such as Ebola;

category B   agents have a similar potential for large-scale dissemination but generally cause less serious illnesses – typhus, brucellosis and food poisoning agents such as *Salmonella* and *E. coli* 0157;

category C   agents include novel infectious diseases which could emerge as future threats.

Furthermore, there is also potential with bioagents to target farm animals and crops, which could cause devastating economic effects. Aflatoxin (a fungal-derived poison or mycotoxin) is a serious human carcinogen and has been identified as a potential biological weapon for food and water contamination.

The production of most of these microorganisms is relatively straightforward when suitable fermentation equipment is available together with the appropriate containment facilities. Final delivery of the microorganism can be problematic for large-scale biowarfare. The most appropriate means of dispersal would be as an aerosol or by contaminating food or water supplies at a local level. The quite serious potential of this new aspect of bioterrorism has created considerable concern in public health authorities. Questions arise as to how quickly these bioweapons can be identified and what form of rapid treatment can be administered. Massive stockpiles of appropriate vaccines and antibiotics must be set in motion, as has already taken place in the USA. Already, the USA has allocated massive funds to research on bioweaponry.

14

Public perception of biotechnology: genetic engineering – safety, social, moral and ethical considerations

14.1   Introduction

While modern biotechnology may be considered as one of the main economic development forces for the twenty-first century, it equally presents far-reaching legal, moral and ethical implications for society. Central to the application of biotechnological techniques to a wide range of industries is gene technology – a controversial and emotive subject.

In the industrialised world, public policy makers on biotechnology have been influenced by the concerted interests of governments, industries, academia and environmental groups. Nationally and internationally, such policies are being developed within a climate of tension and conflicting aims. Central to most of these debates is the single main issue – should regulation be dependent on the characteristics of the products modified by recombinant DNA (rDNA) technology or on the use of the rDNA technology *per se*? The product-versus-process debate has continued for many years and exposes conflicting views on what should represent public policies on new technology development. What is public interest? Should this be left to the scientists and technologists to decide or should the 'public' become part of such decision-making processes? The many crucial decisions to be made will affect the future of humanity and the planet's natural resources. Such decisions should be based on the best scientific information in order to allow effective choices for policy options.

The outcome of these new biotechnological innovations will be most apparent in medicine, agriculture/food and the environment. That the public have a high regard for biomedical research and new therapeutics (recombinant insulin, DNA probes, etc.) is now well recognised. However, public support for agriculture/food developments is less evident, in part because in the developed world food is abundant and cheap, but also because high-profile personalities, and professional pressure groups, have cynically manipulated public concerns about food safety, e.g. aggressively attacking bovine somatotropin (BST) while studiously avoiding genetically engineered chymosin for cheese making.

A dominant feature of public perception of biotechnology is the extraordinarily low and naive public understanding of the genetic basis of life and evolution.

Does public concern really exist or is it largely the manifestation of a well-orchestrated and genuine lobby of knowledgeable opponents? Does genetic engineering get a biased press coverage, e.g. 'Frankenstein foods'? Luddite activists who trample and destroy legitimate field experiments for controllled scientific research into the safety and potential of genetically modified plants should be punished, not applauded, for their nonsensical and destructive behaviour.

It does appear that new biotechnology provokes a variety of views within the public that have not been apparent with many other new technologies. Opinions are influenced by nationality, religion, ethics, morality and knowledge of the core sciences; risk assessment is seldom considered by opponents. Clearly, there is a plurality of views that must be accommodated if democratic decisions are to be made. The need for public education is paramount.

It is important to note that, after hundreds of thousands of studies involving rDNA and the development of many medically useful products used in millions of patients a year, the safety of humans, animals and the environment has been maintained. This clearly demonstrates that high levels of safety and control are being practised by the exponents of new biotechnology.

Some of the main public issues concerning rDNA technology will be examined in some detail.

14.2   Release of genetically manipulated organisms into the environment

In the 1970s, when genetic engineering experiments with microorganisms were first being developed, many molecular biologists believed that the process was unsafe and that manipulated microorganisms should be strictly contained and prevented from release to the environment. The fundamental fear was, and with many still is, that genetically engineered microorganisms could escape from the laboratory into the environment with unpredictable and perhaps catastrophic consequences. It was believed that such released microorganisms could 'upset the balance of nature' or that 'foreign DNA' in the new microorganism could alter its metabolic activity in unpredictable and undesirable ways.

In response to these concerns, guidelines were established to ensure safe working practices and levels of containment based on potential hazards (Chapters 3, 13). However, with time and increased technical awareness, many of these regulations have been progressively relaxed with recognised low-risk systems. Many important medical products, such as insulin and human growth hormone and some industrial enzymes, are manufactured in large-scale containment fermentation processes that involve specific genetically manipulated microorganisms (Chapters 5, 8). The final products from these processes are free of the genetically manipulated host organism and, therefore, do not constitute a release problem. Such systems work well and, to date, there have been no health or environmental problems resulting from their operation. Quite recently, rennet (chymosin) for cheese manufacture has been produced from genetically manipulated microorganisms. An honest, open marketing strategy has shown no adverse public opposition to the final cheese product.

In these previous examples, the manipulated organism was not subject to release and remained within the manufacturing site to be correctly disposed of. However, recombinant microorganisms are now being considered for deliberate release into the environment where they cannot be contained, e.g. biological control, inoculants in agriculture, live vaccines, bioremediation, baker's and brewer's yeast. In addition, we are now witnessing the moving out, in increasing numbers, of recombinant plants from research laboratories and the containment greenhouses and test-plots to the fields and greenhouses of the farmer and large commercial horticulture grower.

What are the dangers associated with environmental release of recombinant organisms? Are they real or mostly imagined? Science fiction writing abounds with stories of deadly microorganisms or plants, e.g. *The Andromeda Strain* and *The Day of the Triffids*, arriving from outer space, enveloping and destroying the human population or the biosphere. Those who oppose the use of recombinant techniques have grasped onto this fiction and have passionately striven to draw comparisons with the release of genetically manipulated organisms.

Increased pathogenicity of microorganisms or microbial ability to destroy essential raw materials are often cited as potential problems of genetically manipulated microorganisms. Pathogenicity is in itself a complex multifactorial process and it is most unlikely that it will be introduced into a previously safe microorganism by a simple gene insertion. Organisms with any possibility of unusual pathogenicity will never be permitted to be used. Where microorganisms are released to be used for biocontrol of, for example, insects, care must be taken that they will not influence other life forms. The use of a recombinant rabies vaccine in baits in Belgium has significantly reduced the level of rabies in wild animals. The public were informed and, in general, approved this worthwhile use of the technology.

All releases into the environment are being carefully monitored and recorded. A major aspect will be to understand how recombinant microorganisms survive and multiply in the environment. Will the recombinant microorganism remain stable or revert back to the original form? And will there be exchange of the recombinant genetic material with other microorganisms? Soil microorganisms are very promiscuous but there is little firm evidence on how much genetic exchange takes place. Much ecological monitoring of microorganisms is now taking place and new methods are being developed. Ecological microbial communities are dynamic systems – neither closed to invasion nor robust in the face of all perturbations. How newly released organisms react to, and interact with, such complex microbial communities will be a major challenge to the microbial ecologist. At present, all new releases of genetically modified microorganisms are considered by expert committees on a case-by-case evaluation. As the information base builds up, it becomes easier to judge new applications. It must be noted that there have been no adverse effects recorded, from the examples so far, for genetically modified microorganisms released into the environment.

Recombinant DNA technology is now being extensively used to improve specific characteristics of plants used for commercial food production. Most of these crops consequently must be grown on a large scale in the open environment to achieve commercial success. A foreseen impediment on the development of manipulated plants for commercial purposes will be the public attitude to such foodstuffs. What are the main concerns that must be addressed to ensure the correct development of this technology to plant agriculture?

The development of transgenic crop varieties is routinely monitored over 2–5 years of field trials to evaluate the performance of the new plants under field conditions. The tasks are normally conducted under strict conditions that prevent the movement of plants and pollen from the test sites. In the USA, since 1987, there have been thousands of field trials with transgenic plants and much valuable information acquired. In general, it would appear that transgenic plants do not look or behave wildly differently from ordinary crop plants. However, there has been some concern expressed that the contained conditions of the field trials do not adequately mirror the real field situations and that some potential environmental hazards could be missed which will only show up after release.

Could transgenic crops move out of the field of cultivation and become weeds? When all commercial crop plants are considered, there are vanishingly few examples where this has happened since such crops require special cultivation practices and are unable to compete with the indigenous wild plant populations. The possibility of gene transfer to compatible wild relatives has been given serious examination. Is it possible that herbicide and pest resistance incorporated into transgenic plants could find its way into other species and increase their 'weediness'? Under normal conditions, gene transfer between close relatives is a very rare and unusual phenomenon and there is little evidence that this will change with transgenic organisms. While such events are theoretically possible, their occurrence would be at such a low frequency that, in practice, the results are of virtually no consequence or concern. However, released transgenic plants will continue to be monitored, to validate these conclusions. Some recombinant genes for pest resistance produce in the plant a product that is toxic to the pest. The possible toxicity of this to humans must always be considered and will be regularly assessed by standard techniques for testing the safety of foods.

14.3   Genetic modification and food uses

Modern biotechnology has its ancestral roots in the early fermentations of foods and beverages which span almost all societies. Since these early times, man has progressively applied selection procedures to encourage beneficial improvements in the individual microorganisms, plants or animals used for food production. While early methods were mainly empirical, the expanding knowledge of genetics allowed a new approach to selective breeding between like species. These, now conventional, genetic techniques, have become accepted worldwide and have not caused any public concern. Genetic engineering is increasingly being applied to many breeding programmes to achieve the same aims as the traditional methods, but offering two main advantages:

(1) the introduction of genes can be controlled with greater prediction and precision than by previous methods.
(2) the introduction of genes into unrelated species is not possible using traditional methods.

The application of genetic engineering to food production is intended to enhance the useful and desirable characteristics of the organisms and to eliminate the undesirable. The overall aim of the food industry, with respect to genetic engineering, will be: to improve the quantity and increase the quality and properties of existing food productions, to produce new products and, of course, to improve financial returns. The consumer has always shown a willingness to pay more for better and more convenient products and to reject products that do not meet their expectations. New biotechnology now offers a major opportunity to tailor food products to public and individual demand.

Previous chapters have highlighted the many *benefits* that genetic engineering might give the producer, including: disease and pest resistance, weed control, animal growth hormones, improved food microorganisms, novel products, improved keeping quality, and 'tailored' products with improved qualities. In contrast, some would consider that there are many potential *risks* associated with these new approaches, including: unintentional transfer of genes into other crops, creations of herbicide-resistant weeds, infringement of plant breeders' rights, increased monoculture, and the undermining of traditional economies. Some believe that it is a technology out of control.

However, a strong prima facie case is increasingly being achieved by the further use of genetic engineering in the manipulation of food organisms for the purpose of improved food production. While the scientific case is strong and persuasive, public perception is somewhat ambivalent. While the public have readily accepted medical products produced from genetically modified organisms (GMOs), they are much less willing to accept such procedures with food. Genetic engineering is seen as 'unnatural' and unnecessary in food production. While scientific opinion is well respected in medical matters by the public, it is often perceived, in matters of food, as purely commercially driven (Table 14.1). People will influence decision making by governments through the ballot box and through the presence of public opinion. Public confidence must be achieved for the success of any new technology.

The safety of the human food supply is based on the concept that there should be a reasonable certainty that no harm will result from its consumption. Foods or food ingredients derived from GMOs must be considered to be as safe as, or safer than, their traditional counterparts before they can be recommended as safe. The most practical approach to the determination of safety is to consider whether the new foods are *substantially equivalent* to analogous conventional food products where they exist and whether their intended use and exposure are relatively similar. Where substantial equivalence is established, no additional safety concerns will normally be expected. Where substantial equivalence is more difficult to establish, then the

Table 14.1. Public attitudes to applications of genetic manipulation in Europe

	% Response		
	Comfortable	Neutral	Uncomfortable
Microbial production of bio-plastics	91	6	3
Cell fusion to improve crops	81	10	10
Curing diseases such as cancer	71	17	9.5
Extension of shelf life of tomatoes	71	11	19
Cleaning up oil slicks	65	20	13
Detoxifying industrial waste	65	20	13
Anti-blood-clotting enzymes produced by rats	65	14	22
Medical research	59	23	15
Making medicines	57	26	13
Making crops to grow in developing countries	54	15	19
	54	15	19
Mastitis-resistant cows by genetic modification of cows	52	16	31
Producing disease-resistant crops	46	29	23
Producing chymosin by microorganisms	43	30	27
Improving crop yields	39	31	29
Using viruses to attack crop pests	32	26	49
Improving milk yields	22	30	47
Cloning prize cattle	7.2	18	72
Changing human physical appearance	4.5	9.5	84
Producing hybrid animals	4.5	12	82
Biological warfare	1.9	2.7	95

identified differences or the new characteristics should be subjected to further safety considerations.

In many countries there are now specialist government-supported committees to check on the safety of GMOs in food production, which examine the technical details for their use or their products destined for the public. In the UK, this is the Advisory Committee on Novel Foods and Processes, with a wide complement of independent, unpaid experts whose opinions and decisions are passed to the food minister, who *then* makes the final official judgement and announcement. The committee is only influenced by the scientific facts and the ultimate safety of the product. Such committees now have, in addition to relevant scientific expertise, strong consumer guidance and expertise on ethics.

While the original concerns about genetically engineered foods were perceived mainly on safety issues, in recent years social, moral and ethical issues have come more to the forefront in decision-making processes.

There is obvious concern that the control of genetically engineered crop plants and their seeds by multinational agrochemical companies, and their need to recoup the high research and investment costs incurred in their development, will imply that only high-technology farmers will be able to carry the cost burden. This will not be true of the farmers in developing countries. Also, herbicide-resistant crops may lead to dependence by farmers on such specific herbicides and, hence, their producing companies.

The concept of *substitutability* will also have dramatic effects on some developing countries. Thus, the development of novel sweeteners (Chapter 11) is already reducing the traditional sugar market for sugar cane and sugar beet, disrupting these economies. In this area, developing countries will most certainly suffer more than the industrialised nations. Increased milk production from fewer cows by the injection of genetically engineered hormones will result in many small farmers in the USA and EEC being put out of business.

Thus, for many aspects of new biotechnology there will be a social price to pay and, particularly in the developing countries, the number of jobs in agriculture will decrease. Different value judgements must be made to reconcile the advantages to society against the disadvantages. The judgements will vary, depending on which side of the poverty line you reside. However, it is encouraging to note that many developing nations are endeavouring to make substantial investments and progress in relevant biotechnology. Technical and financial aid *must* continue to flow to them from the advanced agricultural nations to ensure that they, too, can have the obvious benefits of this technology.

Transgenesis is seen by some as a fundamental breach in natural breeding barriers which nature set up through the process of evolution to prevent genetic interplay between unlike species. In this way the species is seen as 'sacred'. However, in the reductionist viewpoint of many molecular biologists, the gene has become the ultimate unit of life – the gene is merely a unique aggregation of organic molecules (common to all types of cells) available for manipulation. Consequently, they see no ethical problem in transferring genes between species and genera.

It is undoubtedly in the genetic engineering of animals that the 'unnaturalness' of this technology is creating much public unease – for instance, the transfer of a 'human' gene into an animal (Chapter 10), which reflects the fact that the new transgenic organism contains copies of the gene originally obtained from this source. While the transgene has human origin *and* structure, it is not its immediate source. Genes cannot be directly transported from one organism to another but must go through a complicated series of *in vitro* clonings (Chapter 3). This is a series of amplification steps in which the original gene is copied many times during the overall process so that the original genetic material is diluted about 10^{55}. The chance of the original human gene being in the final organism is infinitesimal, or, 'the chances of recovering the original human gene from the transgenic embryo are much less than the chances of recovering a specific drop of water released into the Oceans of the world' (HMSO, 1993). Since the transgenic organism does not contain the actual human gene but, rather, an artificially created copy of the gene, some would consider that the status of the transgene should be considered as that of the new organism. Genes fulfil their biological role only by their activity within the cell of an organism.

An early UK report (by the Committee on the Ethics of Genetic Modification and Food Use, 1993) identified some of the main ethical concerns relating to the food use of certain transgenic organisms:

(1) Transfer of human genes to food animals (e.g. transfer of human gene for factor IX, a protein involved in blood clotting, into sheep (Chapter 8);
(2) Transfer of genes from animals whose flesh is forbidden for use as food by certain religious groups into animals which they normally eat (e.g. pig genes into sheep would offend Jews and Muslims);
(3) Transfer of animal genes into food plants which may be of particular concern to some vegetarians (especially vegans);
(4) Use of organisms containing human genes as animal feed (e.g. yeast modified to produce human proteins of pharmaceutical value and the spent yeast then used as animal feed).

Following consultations covering a wide range of religious beliefs, it was concluded that there were no overriding ethical objections to insist on an absolute prohibition of the use of food products containing copy genes of human origin. However, the report strongly recommended that the use of all ethically sensitive genes in food organisms should be discouraged where alternatives could be found. Products from transgenic organisms containing copy genes that are ethically unacceptable to those groups of the population who are subject to dietary restriction for their religion should be so labelled to ensure choice. The whole aspect of labelling GMO-derived foods is subject to much debate and may eventually be different in different parts of the world. In the not too distant future it is highly possible that all major food organisms will have had some form of genetic engineering in their development and that this could lead to complex labelling criteria. Current discussions between government bodies, industry and consumer organisations will decide the ultimate or realistic extent of labelling required to meet ethical requirements.

Genetic engineering of animals may also arouse severe moral opposition if there are instances of animals suffering as a result of this process. Already there is evidence of animals suffering severe arthritis following application of transgenic growth hormones to improve their meat quality.

While some religious groups exercise strong discrimination of the type of animal that can be eaten, the position can be quite different when considered from a medically derived product (insulin from a pig pancreas) or the transplant of an animal organ. Almost all faiths take the view that preservation of human life is the first priority. Thus, pig-derived insulin can be accepted by a Jew and by a Muslim only with special religious permission. Similarly, a Jew could accept a pig organ transplant if absolutely essential. These contrary positions are supported by the view that the human body can only be violated by oral intake and not by other methods of introduction such as by injection or surgery.

A recent US Institute of Food Technologists' Expert Panel concluded that continued development and use of food rDNA biotechnology provide a number of important benefits to society:

- a more abundant and economical food supply for the world;
- continued improvements in nutritional quality, including foods of unique composition for populations whose diets lack essential nutrients;
- fresh fruit and vegetables with improved shelf life;
- the development of functional foods, vaccines and similar products, which may provide health and medical benefits;
- further improvements in production agriculture through more efficient production practices and increased yields;
- the conversion of non-productive toxic soils, in developing countries, to productive arable land;
- more environmentally friendly agricultural practices through improved pesticides and pesticide-usage practices, less hazardous animal wastes, improved utilisation of land, and reduced need for ecologically sensitive areas such as rainforests.

Furthermore, with respect to a range of environmental and economic concerns about rDNA-biotechnology-derived food products, the panel also reached the following conclusions:

Table 14.2. Areas of public concern in human genome research

Confidentiality of testing and screening results
Scope of genetic testing and screening
Discrimination and stigmatisation
Commercial exploitation of human genome data
Eugenic pressures
Effects of germ-line gene therapies on later generations

From European Federation of Biotechnology (1995).

- New rDNA-biotechnology-derived foods and food products do not inherently present any more serious environmental concerns or unintended toxic properties than those already presented by conventional breeding practices.
- Appropriate testing by technology developers, producers and processors, regulatory agencies and others should be continued for new foods and food products derived from all technologies, including rDNA biotechnology.
- Programmes should be developed to provide the benefits of safe and economical rDNA-biotechnology-derived food products worldwide, including less-developed countries.

14.4 The applications of human genetic research

Several thousand genetic disorders of humans would appear to result from a mutation in single genes, while many others have more complex genetic explanations and even possible interactions with environmental factors (Chapter 8). Results from the Human Genome Project, discussed earlier, are now considered to offer an increased understanding of these fundamental genetic malfunctions and to give, in some cases, hope for alleviation and perhaps cure of the defect. However, paralleling the scientific breakthroughs and deeper understandings of gene mechanisms have come many areas of public concern (Table 14.2).

The major nations now committed to genome projects are also supporting research into the many ethical, legal and social issues that these studies are uncovering. Numerous committees now foster public debate and understanding of these highly complex issues. On the one hand the scientific discoveries could possibly bring much relief to millions of sufferers of genetic diseases, but on the other they give rise to questions of mind-bending implications as to the way forward for the human race.

Genetic testing and screening

Where genetic disorders have previously been observed in families, it is now possible in some cases to carry out pre-natal testing to discover whether the foetus carries the defect. The parents may then be able to sanction an abortion or be better prepared for the needs of the full-term baby. There are obvious concerns that this could result in a wide range of other conditions being selected for termination, e.g. gender and diseases of a minor nature. Soon it may be possible to have a much fuller awareness of an individual's 'genetic portfolio' and possibly to diagnose future medical problems, e.g. heart disease and cancer, and advise treatment well in advance of the onset of the disease. However, would an individual wish to know that they would develop Huntington's disease (presently an untreatable, debilitating and often fatal disease) in 30–40 years' time? It has been suggested that genetic testing and screening should only be carried out with disorders where treatment is available.

Perhaps the most worrying aspect of such genetic testing is the use to which such information could be put by insurance and mortgage institutions. While undoubtedly such financial systems would reduce the risk aspect of their investments, the effects on the individual would be devastating. It is increasingly viewed by ethics' committees that insurance companies should not require, or be allowed access to, an individual's genetic information as a prerequisite for insurance. This may well prove to be an impossible task to monitor and control. It is increasingly becoming apparent that the course of an individual's future is not 'in the stars' but, in reality, in their own genes!

Human gene therapy Gene therapy can be considered from either a somatic or germ-line approach (Chapter 8). From an ethical viewpoint somatic-cell gene therapy involving the insertion of single genes into a patient is really no different from the long-accepted practice of transplants, e.g. hearts and lungs, from other individuals. It is considered that such treatments should be used only to alleviate serious medical disorders and not for non-therapeutic applications. The application of gene therapy could be important to the pharmaceutical industry but it is not yet clear whether it could be sold as an injectable 'product' or be dispensed as a service. Part of the confusion comes from the vast diversity of potential disease applications, ranging from immunotherapeutics to genetic diseases. In either case it will not be a cheap therapy. Somatic gene therapy must remain under close supervision to satisfy medical safety, legal implications and public concerns.

Germ-line gene therapy is presently not being pursued because it is technically extremely difficult and is ethically and socially unacceptable. Interfering with germ cells raises huge problems of eugenics and there must be extensive public debate if it is ever to be used as a meaningful medical technique.

Stem cells – undifferentiated primordial cells – are derived from a single fertilised egg and have the potential to develop into various tissues that can eventually produce different types of organs. It is believed that stem cells could have the potential to develop cures for many diseases, e.g. diabetes and Alzheimer's. Stem cells could also lead the way to therapeutic cloning, with the cloning of organs (kidney, heart, etc.) for transplantation purposes. Sadly, there is much opposition to this area of research on ethical and moral grounds.

Some general conclusions are now appearing from the increased level of discussion of these issues. The public does not accept or reject gene technology as a whole. Parts of it will be welcomed and utilised while other parts will have less, or no, support at all. The biotechnology community must aim to inform, not indoctrinate, the public. The consumers and patients of biotechnology products must be given clear and unequivocable information. A recent EEC 'public perception of biotechnology' meeting ended with the following message to biotechnology companies: 'Provide the information and listen to the public'.

When taking into consideration the scientific complexity of most new biotechnology products and processes, companies must use public relations effectively to provide consumers with adequate information about the advantages and benefits of their products. In this way the public will be able to make informed decisions about them. Similarly, scientists must learn to communicate with the public, be willing to do so, and consider it a duty to do so! The most significant obstacles to the full creative resolution of new biotechnology are not expected to be scientific, economic or indeed environmental but, rather, cultural!

15

Looking to the future

Biotechnology has been shown to be a spectrum of enabling technologies which are increasingly being applied in many aspects of modern society. The applied use of biological systems, especially microorganisms, in such processes as brewing, wine making and cheese production was primarily accomplished in an empirical manner, with the management of these processes seen more as an art rather than a science. In recent times these ancient biotechnological processes have been subjected to rigorous scientific study and analysis, which has largely led to the replacement of traditional empiricism. Better understanding of microbial strain selection, molecular biology and genetics, together with improved bioprocess technology, have yielded major advances in all of the traditional biotechnology industries and will continue to achieve improved quality and safety together with cost-effectiveness.

A central feature of new biotechnological advances derives from an increasing understanding of the mechanisms of life and how these will eventually transform human lives as well as give a deeper appreciation of agriculture, aquaculture, forestry and the biological environment. The ability to select and manipulate genetic material within and outwith species has permitted unprecedented opportunities to alter life forms for the benefit of society. The successful sequencing of the human and other genomes is the beginning of a new scientific period of discovery. However, rather than genomic sequences being an end in themselves, it is but the beginning of scientific study to put the information into context with regard to the biological significance to the organism. Currently, sequence data have been used to identify species, to derive evolutionary linkages and to study the basis of organism diversity.

Many molecular biologists have postulated that a genetic or DNA sequence analysis of an individual could be predictive of future disease occurrence, e.g. cardiovascular disease, cancer and Alzheimer's disease. This has generated much interest, especially with insurance companies. However, to rely on sequence analysis alone would be insufficient since this would not take into consideration all the multivarious adaptive systems of the living organism as well as the environmental input threshold on an individual's lifespan. However, new microarray technology, where thousands of single-nucleotide polymorphisms can be analysed, together with advances in proteomics may well give a meaningful patient read-out on potential susceptibility and early diagnosis of an impending problem, allowing much earlier medical or lifestyle intervention. Recombinant DNA technology of mammalian cell cultures has produced many recombinant proteins, e.g. insulin and recombinant vaccines, which are now bringing considerable medical benefit to a wide range of human diseases. Undoubtedly, there will be continued research and application in this area.

The present applications of genetic engineering technology to the life sciences, through apparently revolutionary techniques, are indeed nothing to what will evolve in the future. The further implementation of genomics and proteomics will allow a much deeper understanding of the biology of molecules, cells and whole organisms. Doctors and patients will have much to gain from the outcome of these studies. Much will be learned about human individuality and how these findings could influence individual health and disease susceptibility.

Plant-based genetic engineering did not really start until the early 1980s with the development of the Ti plasmid of *Agrobacterium tumifaciens*, which has allowed the introduction of simple genetic constructs into most of the important crop plants. These processes are now relatively routine, and the changes made within the plants have been so slight that it requires highly sophisticated biochemical assays to distinguish genetically modified varieties from their predecessors. Notwithstanding the large and growing body of evidence that the application of plant genetic engineering is safe and that development has always been applied responsibly and safely, there has been a small but highly organised and vociferous opposition to the application of the technology.

The application of any new technology is often fraught with public misconception and mistrust of scientific opinion. No technology can ever be free of risk and, in our present affluent developed world, perfection is now the expectation. Irresponsible media 'experts' (often with no scientific experience) lead the public to expect zero impact and risk from the new technological innovations of plant genetic engineering, and if any slight deficiency – real or imagined – is detected, they will propose the complete condemnation of the practice. The demand for moratoria or outright banning of GM food products, particularly in Europe, has its origins in inflammatory and unscientific phrases such as 'biological pollution' and 'Frankenstein food' and erroneous comparisons made with BSE, foot and mouth disease and nuclear power plants. The scientific community involved in GM food studies has shown a level of caution that has been lacking in most other new technologies. The basic work is routine and well established. There are few, if any, real risks associated with genetic engineering of crop plants that could in any way compete with the hazards that society presently accepts in order to uphold current ways of life, e.g. transport, smoking, alcohol, and many others.

In 2001, the estimated global commitment to GM crops was about 53 million hectares being grown by 5.5 million farmers. The USA grew 68% of the total, followed by Argentina (22%), Canada (6%) and China (3%). Many other countries, including Bulgaria, Uruguay, Indonesia, Brazil and Mexico, are now in the early stages of growing transgenic crops. There is increasing evidence that GM crops are giving significant yield increases, savings for growers, and pesticide-use reductions in both developed and developing countries. Unfortunately, Europe will continue to suffer bureaucratic/political constraints on the legislation of GM crops. There is clearly no scientific basis or thinking that can justify this luddite approach.

At present, single gene transfers are the basis of current plant genetic engineering. However, current studies on plant genomes are now identifying sets of genes that influence plant architecture, such as root thickness and area, leaf size and shape, which will be of great value to plant breeders for increasing yields without increasing acreage. At the present time many of the applications of GM plant technology have benefited the farmer rather than the consumer. However, in the near future this trend will change, with more emphasis being given to human and animal nutrition.

Our present knowledge of human nutrition is now well defined at a population level and food processors can now compensate for most nutrient imbalances in staple foods by adding supplements such as essential amino acids and vitamins. In the future the plant breeder and the farmer may well be able to manipulate crop plants to much more exact nutritional requirements. Rice is deficient in vitamin A, resulting in blindness in children in many developing communities where it is a dietary staple. The development of GM rice strains with raised levels of vitamin A and iron has now been achieved and will be of immense nutritional value, especially to populations in developing countries. All patent rights on this production in the developing world have been waived by the scientists and companies involved. Future GM plant technology will facilitate in-plant formulation of nutrients for human consumption.

Since plant crops such as cereals are the basis of most farmed animal diets, it can be anticipated that most crops will be engineered to suit the exact nutritional requirements of individual animal species, i.e. cattle, pigs and poultry.

The new aspects of biotechnology, such as transgenic plants and animals, recombinant proteins and vaccines, will bring huge benefits to mankind but not without generating concern in some sections of the population. Biotechnologists, in general, stand accused of not communicating with the lay public, largely because the scientists have mostly been unable or unwilling to take the time to explain in simple, understandable language the basic principles of the science involved. They must also be more circumspect in the claims made for the future outcome of their studies. There are still vast areas of biological knowledge that must be deciphered before most speculative projects can be achieved. Also, the time-scale for accomplishment must also be more realistic.

The ethical and moral issues raised by some aspects of new biotechnology must be addressed by continued open discussion and informed communication. Scare stories generate more public interest than honest reassuring facts. Furthermore, and a direct criticism of the present educational system, most of the population are ignorant of even simple biological facts and, naturally, find the complexity of genetic engineering bewildering and threatening.

In practice, the majority of products to be derived from biotechnology will be recognisable extensions of existing ones or will stem from improvements in production. Minor improvements in processes by many of these new technologies may not be highly newsworthy but will help to give producer companies a competitive edge. The history of biotechnology shows how intimate the interplay must be between industry and academia to maintain the creative effort to generate new products and to expand their scope, profitability and social benefits.

Although there is now a vast reservoir of relevant biological and engineering knowledge and expertise waiting to be put into productive biotechnological use, the eventual rate of application will be determined not primarily by science and technology but, rather, by many other equally important factors such as industrial investment policies, the establishment of market needs, the economics of the marketing skills needed to introduce new products into commercial use and, above all, how the public perceive this new range of innovative technologies.

Biotechnology will play a major role in the continued search for solutions to the many problems that will affect the society of tomorrow, namely health, food supply and a safe biological environment. Continued scientific research will be paramount to achieving these ends. However, as Louis Pasteur commented on the inexorable nature of scientific studies:

> *As the circle of light increases, so too does the circumference of darkness.*

Glossary

Activated sludge process   Aerobic sewage treatment process using aerobic microorganisms present in sewage sludge to break down organic matter in sewage.

Aerated pile   Microbial composition of organic waste matter where the wastes are heaped in piles and forced aeration supplies oxygen.

Aerobic   Living or acting only in the presence of oxygen.

Amino acids   The building blocks of proteins.

Anaerobe   Microorganisms that can grow and multiply in the absence of oxygen.

Anaerobic digestion   A microbial fermentation of organic matter to methane and CO_2 which occurs in near absence of air; a sewage treatment process.

Antibiotic   A specific type of chemical substance that is used to fight microbial infections, usually in humans or animals. Most antibiotics are produced by microorganisms. Semi-synthetic antibiotics are natural antibiotics that have been modified chemically.

Antibody   A protein produced by the immune system on exposure to a specific antigen, characterised by specific reactivity with its complementary antigen.

Antigen   A molecule introduced into an organism and recognised as a foreign material, resulting in the elicitation of antibody production (immune response) directed specifically against the foreign molecule.

Antisense genes   Genes in which the mirror image of the normal nucleotide base sequences is inserted, preventing expression of the natural genes.

Ascites   Liquid accumulation in the peritoneal cavity, widely used as a method for propagating hybridoma cells for monoclonal antibody formation.

Bacteriophage   A virus that multiplies in bacteria.

Biological oxygen demand (BOD)   The oxygen used in meeting the metabolic needs of aerobic organisms in water containing organic compounds.

Biomass   All organic matter that derives from the photosynthetic conversion of solar energy.

Bioreactor (fermenter)   Containment system for fermentation purposes.

Biosensor   An electronic device that uses biological molecules to detect specific compounds.

Bovine somatotropin   Growth hormone that can be produced by recombinant DNA technology and used to increase the milk yield by cows.

Callus   Plant cells that are capable of repeated cell division and growth.

Cell line   Cells that acquire the ability to multiply indefinitely *in vitro*.

Chromosome   A thread of DNA in the nucleus which carries genetic inheritance.

Chymosin   An enzyme used to clot milk, which is used in the manufacture of cheese.

Clone   A collection of genetically identical cells or organisms derived from a common ancestor; all members of the clone have identical genetic composition.

Conjugation   The transfer of genetic material from one cell to another by cell-to-cell contact.

Continuous fermentation   A fermentation process that can run for long periods, in which raw materials are supplied and products and microorganisms are removed continuously.

DNA probes   Isolated single DNA strands used to detect the presence of the complementary (opposite) strands, and used as very sensitive biological detectors.

Downstream processing   Separation and purification of product(s) from a fermentation process.

Embryo transfer   Implementation of embryos from donor animals or generated by *in vitro* fertilisation into the uteri of recipient animals.

Enzyme   A class of proteins that control biological reactions.

Enzyme bioreactor   A reactor in which a chemical conversion reaction is catalysed by an enzyme.

Fermentation   The process by which microorganisms turn raw materials such as glucose into products such as alcohol.

Gene   A unit of heredity; a segment of DNA coding for a specific protein.

Gene transfer   The use of genetic or physical manipulations to introduce foreign genes into host cells to achieve desired characteristics in progeny.

Genetic engineering   Technologies, including DNA technologies, used to isolate genes from an organism, manipulate them in the laboratory, and insert them into another cell system.

Genome   The genetic endowment of an organism or individual that resides with the nucleic acids of the chromosomes.

Hybridoma   A unique fused cell which produces quantities of a specific antibody, and reproduces endlessly.

Immobilised enzyme   An enzyme which is physically defined or localised in a defined region, enabling it to be re-used in a continuous process.

Ligase enzyme   An enzyme used by genetic engineers to join cut ends of DNA strands.

Lignocellulose   The composition of woody biomass, including lignin and cellulose.

Metabolite   A product of biochemical activity.

Micropropagation   The use of small pieces of tissue, such as meristem, grown in culture to produce large numbers of plants.

Monoclonal antibody   An antibody derived from a single source or cone of cells which recognises only one kind of antigen.

Mutation   Stable changes of a gene inherited on reproduction.

Particle gun bombardment   A method of introducing DNA into a host plant cell. It involves precipitating DNA onto microscopic particles or projectiles. The particles are then accelerated and penetrate the plant cells, depositing DNA.

Plasmid   A loop of DNA found in bacteria and some other organisms, e.g. yeasts, that carries non-essential genes and replicates independently of the chromosomes.

Polymerase chain reaction (PCR)   The action of an enzyme (polymerase) in producing many copies of a polynucleotide sequence of DNA.

Promoter sequence   A regulatory DNA sequence that initiates the expression of a gene.

Proteins   A large molecule consisting of amino acids, and the product of genes.

Protein engineering   Generating proteins with subtly modified structures, conferring properties such as higher catalytic specificity or thermal stability.

Proteome   The collective body of proteins made within an organism's cells and tissues.

Protoplast   A microbial or plant cell whose wall has been removed so that the cell assumes a spherical shape.

Recombinant DNA   The hybrid DNA produced by joining pieces of DNA from different organisms.

Restriction enzyme   An enzyme used by molecular biologists to cut through DNA at specific points.

Restriction fragment length polymorphism (RFLP)   Fragments of differing lengths of DNA that are produced by cutting DNA with restriction enzymes.

Scale-up   The expansion of laboratory experiments to full-sized industrial processes.

Single cell protein   Cells or protein extracts of microorganisms grown in large quantities for use as human or animal protein supplements.

Somaclonal variation   Genetic variation produced from the culture of plant cells from a pure breeding strain.

Splicing   Gene splicing, or manipulation, the object of which is to attach one DNA molecule to another.

Tissue culture   A process whereby individual cells, or clumps of plant or animal tissue, are grown artificially.

Transduction   The transfer of bacterial genes from one bacterium to another by a virus (bacteriophage).

Transformation   The acquisition of new genetic markers by the incorporation of added DNA.

Transgenic organism   An animal, plant or microorganism where hereditary DNA has been augmented by the addition of DNA from a source other than parental germ plasm.

Vector   A vehicle for transferring DNA from one cell to another.

Further reading

New developments in biotechnology are covered in many journals; in particular, reference should be made regularly to *Bio/Technology* (ISSN-22X), Nature Publishing Co., New York.

Advisory Committee on Science and Technology. *Developments in Biotechnology*. London: HMSO, 1990.

Alexander, H. Biodegradation of chemicals of environmental concern. *Science* **211** (1981), 132–8.

Angold, R., Beech, G. and Taggart, J. *Food Biotechnology*. Cambridge: Cambridge University Press, 1989.

Asenjo, J. A. (ed.). *Separation Processes in Biotechnology*. New York: Marcel Dekker, 1990.

Atlas, R. and Bartha, R. *Microbial Ecology, 3rd edn*. Wokingham, UK: Benjamin/Cummings Publishing Co. 1983.

Bains, W. and Evans, C. The business of biotechnology. In *Basic Biotechnology*, 2nd edn, ed. C. Ratledge and B. Kristiansen. Cambridge: Cambridge University Press, 2001, pp. 255–79.

Beddey, R. 'Green' energy from sugar cane. *Chemistry & Industry*, **May** (1993), 355–8.

Beringer, J. E. Is there a future for GMOs? *Biologist* **42** (2000), 81–4.

Beringer, J. E. and Bale, M. J. Releasing genetically modified microorganisms to the environment. *Biologist* **39** (1992), 49–51.

Berry, D. Yeast matters. *Biologist* **46** (1999), 211–14.

Bienz-Tadmor, B. Biopharmaceuticals go to market: patterns of world-wide development. *Bio/Technology* **11** (1993), 168–71.

BIOTOL (Biotechnology by Open Learning). A series of books. Oxford: Butterworth (Heinemann Ltd).

Bio-Wise. *Industrial Solid Waste Treatment: A Review of Composting/Technology*. Bio-Wise, PO Box 83, Didcot, Oxfordshire OX11 0BR, 2001.

Bolin, F. Levelling land mines with biotechnology. *Nature Biotechnology* **17** (1999), 732.

Bremner, C. and Conner, J. International Initiative in Biotechnology for Developing Country Agriculture: Promises and Problems. Paris: OECD, 1994.

British Medical Association. *Our Genetic Future: the Science and Ethics of Gene Technology*. Oxford: Oxford University Press, 1992.

Brooks, R., Anderson, C., Stewart, R. and Robinson, B. Phytomining: growing a crop of a metal. *Biologist* **46** (1999), 201–5.

Brown, T. A. *Essential Molecular Biology*. Oxford: IRL Press, 1991.

Budd, R. *The Uses of Life: A History of Biotechnology*. New York: Cambridge University Press, 1993.

Bull, A. T. Clean technology: industry and environment – a viable partnership. *Biologist* **47** (2003), 61–4.

Bull, A. T., Holt, G. and Lilly, M. D. *Biotechnology: International Trends and Perspectives*. Paris: OECD, 1982.

Campbell-Platt, G. *Fermented Foods of the World: A Dictionary and Guide*. London: Butterworth, 1989.

Cash, P. Proteomics: the protein revolution. *Biologist* **49** (2002), 58–62.

Castro-Rios, A. Human rights in the world of genetic revolution. *Human Reproduction and Genetic Ethics* **5** (1999), 26–30.

Chang, S.-T. World production of cultivated edible and medicinal mushrooms in 1997. *International Journal of Medicinal Mushrooms* **1** (1999), 291–300.

Chemistry & Industry. Special Issue 'Environmental Technology', June, No. 11, 1994.

Davies, J. E. and Demain, A. L. *Manual of Industrial Microbiology and Biotechnology*, *2nd edn*. Washington DC: America Society of Microbiology, 1999.

de Chadarevian, S. *Designs for Life: Molecular Biology after World War II*. Cambridge: Cambridge University Press, 2002, p. 423.

Della-Cioppa, G. and Callan, M. Sex, lies and herbicides. *Nature Biotechnology* **18** (2000), 241.

Desmorescaux, P. and Hodgson, J. Building a common future. *Nature Biotechnology* **17** (1999), BVI.

Durrant, J. R., Evans, G. A. and Thomas, G. P. The public understanding of science. *Nature* **340** (1989), 11–14.

Eggeling, L., Pfefferle, W. and Sahm, H. (2001). Amino acids. In *Basic Biotechnology*, ed. C. Ratledge and B. Kristiansen. Cambridge: Cambridge University Press, pp. 281–304.

European Federation of Biotechnology (EFB). Biotechnology in foods and drinks. Briefing Paper 2. Task Group on Public Perceptions of Biotechnology. Holland: EFB, 1994.

  The Application of Human Genetic Research. Briefing Paper 3. Task Group on Public Perceptions of Biotechnology. Holland: EFB, 1995.

Environmental Biotechnology. Holland: EFB, 1999.
http://www.kluyver.stm.tudelft.nl/ef6/hom.htm.

Fincham, J. R. G. and Ravetz, J. R. *Genetically Engineered Organisms – Risks and Benefits*. Buckingham: Open University Press, 1991.

Flavell, R. B. Agriculture: a path of experiment and change. *Nature Biotechnology* **17** suppl. (1999), 7–8.

Forster, C. F. *Biotechnology and Waste-Water Treatment*. Cambridge Studies in Biotechnology 2. Cambridge: Cambridge University Press, 1985.

Fry, J. C. and Day, M. (eds.). *Release of Genetically Engineered and Other Microorganisms*. Cambridge: Cambridge University Press, 1993.

Godfrey, T. and Reichelt, J. *Industrial Enzymology. The Application of Enzymes in Industry*. London: Macmillan, 1983.

Golub, E. *The Limits of Medicine: How Science Shapes Our Hope for the Cure*. New York: Time Books, 1994.

The constant presence of death. *Bio/Technology* **13** (1995), 191–2.

Graham, A. A haystack of needles: applying the polymerase chain reaction. *Chemistry & Industry* **October** (1994), 718–21.

Grainger, J. and Madden, D. The polymerase chain reaction: turning needles into haystacks. *Biologist* **40** (1993), 197–200.

Gray, J. *The Genetic Engineer and Biotechnologist*. Swansea: GB Biotechnology Ltd, 1990.

Guarraia, L. J., Ryse, R. S., Godown, R. D. and Agar, B. Genetic engineering: existing safeguards. *Our Planet* **6** (1994), 42–5.

Hacking, A. J. *Economic Aspects of Biotechnology*. Cambridge Studies in Biotechnology 3. Cambridge: Cambridge University Press, 1986.

Hammond, S. M. and Lambert, P. A. *Antibiotics and Antimicrobial Action*. Studies in Biology, No. 90. London: Edward Arnold, 1978.

Harris, B. Magic bullets. *Chemistry & Industry*, **September** (1991), 656–9.

Harris, F., Chatfield, L. and Phoenix, D. A. The gene genie. *Biologist* **49** (2002), 25–8.

Higgins, I. J., Best, D. J. and Jones, J. *Biotechnology, Principles and Applications*. Oxford: Blackwell Scientific Publications, 1985.

Hodgson, J. Biosafety rules get thumbs up. *Nature Biotechnology* **18** (2000a), 253.
Crystal-gazing – the new biotechnologies. *Nature Biotechnology* **18** (2000b), 29–31.

Jacobsson, S., Jamison, A. and Rothman, H. *The Biotechnology Challenge*. Cambridge: Cambridge University Press, 1986.

Jaroff, L. Happy birthday double helix. *Time Magazine*, March 15 (1993), 50–8.

Johnson, K. Prospects for gene therapy. *Chemistry and Industry* (1991), 644–6.

Jones, H. and Wiley, P. The double helix. *Biologist* **50** (2003), 53–7.

King, P. P. Biotechnology: an industrial view. *Journal of Chemical Technology and Biotechnology* **32** (1982), 2–8.

Krijgsman, J. *Production Recovery in Bioprocess Technology*. BIOTOL Series. Oxford: Butterworth Heinemann, 1992.

Kristiansen, K. and Chamberlain, H. (1983). Fermenter systems. In *The Filamentous Fungi, Vol. 4*, ed. Smith, J. E., Berry, D. R. and Kristiansen, B. London: Edward Arnold, pp. 48–61.

Lappé, M. and Bailey, B. *Against the Grain. Genetic Transformation of Global Agriculture*. Earthscan Publications, 1999.

Marshall, A. The insects are coming. *Nature Biotechnology* **16** (1998), 530–3.

McCormick, D. K. First words, last words. *Bio/Technology* **14** (1996), 224.

Mittwoch, U. 'Clone': the history of a euphonious scientific term. *Medical History* **46** (2002), 381–402.

Morgan, P. *Biotechnology and Oil Spills*. Shell Centre London SE1 7NA: Group Public Affairs, Shell Industrial Petroleum Company Ltd., 1991.

Moser, A. Sustainable biotechnology development: from high tech to eco-tech. *Acta Biotechnology* **12** (1994), 2–6.

Office of Technology Assessment. *Commercial Biotechnology: An International Analysis*. Washington DC: US Congress, 1984.
 Bioremediation for Marine Oil Spills. Washington DC: US Congress, 1991.

Old, R. W. and Primrose, S. B. *Principles of Gene Manipulations – An Introduction to Genetic Engineering*. Oxford: Blackwell Scientific Publications, 1990.

Organisation for Economic Cooperation and Development (OECD). *Biotechnology: Economic and Wider Impacts*. Paris: OECD, 1989.
 Biotechnology, Agriculture and Food. Paris: OECD, 1992.
 Safety Evaluation of Foods Derived by Modern Biotechnology. Paris: OECD, 1993.
 Biotechnology for Clean Industrial Products and Processes: Towards Industrial Sustainability. Paris: OECD, 1998.

Owen, M. R. L., Gandecha, A., Cockburn, B. and Whitelaw, G. C. The expression of antibiotics in plants. *Chemistry & Industry*, **June** (1992), 406–8.

Parekh, R. Proteomics and molecular medicine. *Nature Biotechnology* **17** (1999), 19–20.

Pennington, H. Millennium bugs. *Biologist* **47** (2000), 93–5.

Powell, W. and Hillman, J. R. *Opportunities and Problems in Plant Biotechnology*. Edinburgh: Proceedings of the Royal Society of Edinburgh, 1992, p. 182.

Ratledge, C. and Kristiansen, B. (eds). *Basic Biotechnology*. Cambridge: Cambridge University Press (contains a wide selection of relevant chapters).

Rexroad, C. E. Transgenic livestock in agriculture and medicine. *Chemistry & Industry*, **April** (1995), 372–5.

Roberts, S. M., Turner, N. T., Willets, A. and Turner, M. K. *Introduction to Biocatalysis using Whole Enzymes and Microorganisms*. Cambridge: Cambridge University Press, 1995.

Robinson, C. Making forest biotechnology a commercial reality. *Nature Biotechnology* **17** (1999), 27–30.

Salamini, F. North–South innovation transfer. *Nature Biotechnology* **17** suppl. (1999), 11–12.

Scientific American. *Industrial Microbiology and the Advent of Genetic Engineering*. A Scientific American Book. New York: W. H. Freeman & Co., 1981.

Slesser, M. and Lewis, C. *Biological Energy Reserves*. London: E & F. M. Spon, 1979.

Smith, J. E. *Biotechnology Principles*. Aspects of Microbiology II. Holland: Van Nostrand Reinhold, 1985.

Smith, J. E., Rowan, N. J. and Sullivan, R. Medicinal mushrooms: a rapidly developing area of biotechnology for cancer therapy and other bioactivities. *Biotechnology Letters* **24** (2002), 1839–45.

Snell, N. Bioterrorism today. *Biologist* **49** (2002), 140.

Speir, R. E. (ed.). *The Encyclopaedia of Cell Technology*. New York: John Wiley, 2002.

Spencer, R. and Lightfoot, N. Preparedness and response to bioterrorism. *Journal of Infection* **43** (2001), 104–10.

Staat, F. and Vallet, E. Vegetable oil methyl ester as a diesel substitute. *Chemistry & Industry*, **November** (1994), 863–5.

Stanbury, P. F. and Whitaker, A. *Principles of Fermentation Technology*. Oxford: Pergamon Press, 1984.

Steinbuerg, F. M. and Raso, J. Biotech pharmaceuticals and biotherapy: an overview. *Journal of Pharmacy and Pharmaceutical Science* **1** (1998), 48–59.

Stewart, C. N. (2003). *Transgenic Plants: Current Innovations and Future Trends*. Norfolk: Horizon Press, p. 297.

The Royal Society. *Transgenic Plants and World Agriculture*. London: The Royal Society, 2000, www.royalsoc.ac.uk.

  Genetically Modified Plants for Food Use and Human Health – An Update. London: The Royal Society, 2002, www.royalsoc.ac.uk

Walgate, R. *Miracle or Menace: Biotechnology and the Third World*. London: The Panos Institute, 1990.

Waste Management and Recycling International. Sterling Publications Ltd., 86–88 Edgware Road, London W2 2YW, 1994.

Watson, J. S. and Tooze, J. *The DNA Story*. New York: W. H. Freeman & Co., 1981.

Wells, D. A. and Herron, L. L. Automated sample preparation for genomics. *PharmaGenomics* **2** (2002), 52–5.

Williamson, R. and Kampmann, D. Gene therapy – the great debate. *Human Reproduction and Genetic Ethics* **2** (1998), 25–8.

Wood, B. J. B. (ed.). *The Microbiology of Fermented Foods, Vols 1 and 2*, 2nd edn. London: Elsevier Applied Science Publishers, 1998.

Wymer, P. Making sense of biosensors. NCBE Newsletter. Reading: Reading University, 1990.

Yanchinski, S. and Sasaki, M. *Setting Genes to Work: The Industrial Era of Biotechnology*. New York: Viking, 1985.

Yokotsuka, T. Fermented protein foods in the Orient, with emphasis on shoyu and miso in Japan. In *Microbiology of Fermented Foods, Vol. 1*, ed. B. J. B. Wood. London: Elsevier Applied Science Publishers, 1985, pp. 351–415.

Index